Nursing for Public Health
Population-based Care

Edited by

Pauline M Craig MSc BSc RGN HV
Health Visitor/Senior Health Promotion Officer,
Greater Glasgow Health Board, UK

Grace M Lindsay PhD MN BSc(Hons) RGN RM
Lecturer, Nursing and Midwifery School, University of Glasgow, UK

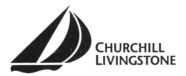

CHURCHILL
LIVINGSTONE

EDINBURGH LONDON NEW YORK PHILADELPHIA ST LOUIS SYDNEY TORONTO 2000

CHURCHILL LIVINGSTONE
An imprint of Harcourt Publishers Limited

© Harcourt Publishers Limited 2000

⤶ is a registered trademark of Harcourt Publishers Limited

First published 2000

0 443 05942 X

British Library Cataloguing in Publication Data
A catalogue record for this book is available from the British Library

Library of Congress Cataloging in Publication Data
A catalog record for this book is available from the Library of Congress

Note
Medical knowledge is constantly changing. As new information becomes available, changes in treatment, procedures, equipment and the use of drugs become necessary. The editors and the publishers have, as far as it is possible, taken care to ensure that the information given in this text is accurate and up to date. However, readers are strongly advised to confirm that the information, especially with regard to drug usage, complies with the latest legislation and standards of practice.

SMC

The
publisher's
policy is to use
**paper manufactured
from sustainable forests**

Printed in China

Contents

Contributors

Pauline Craig
Health Visitor/Senior Health Promotion Officer,
Greater Glasgow Health Board, Glasgow

Yvonne Dalziel
Community Development Programme Manager,
Lothian Primary Care NHS Trust Edinburgh

Di Douglas
Clinical Effectiveness Facilitator,
The State Hospital, Carstairs

Carol Fraser
Senior Public Health Infection Control Advisor,
Lothian Health, Edinburgh

Rosie Ilett
Coordinator, Centre for Women's Health, Glasgow

Grace Lindsay
Lecturer, Nursing and Midwifery Studies,
University of Glasgow, Glasgow

Emma McIntosh
Research Fellow, Health Economics Research Unit,
University of Aberdeen, Aberdeen

Jean B McIntosh
Professor, Nursing Studies, Glasgow Caledonian University, Glasgow

Kate Munro
Training Officer, Centre for Women's Health, Glasgow

Stephen Peckham
Senior Lecturer in Social Policy, Department of Sociology,
Oxford Brookes University, Oxford

Mandy Ryan
MRC Senior Fellow, Health Economics Research Unit,
University of Aberdeen, Aberdeen

Joan Sneddon
Senior Nursing Advisor (Infection Control),
Lanarkshire Health Board, Hamilton

Suzie Stewart
Department of Public Health, University of Glasgow, Glasgow

Pat Taylor
Public Health Alliance, Birmingham

Pat Turton
Director of Education, Bristol Cancer Help Centre, Bristol

Robert West
Reader, Department of Public Health,
University of Wales College of Medicine, Cardiff

John Wormersley
Consultant in Public Health, Department of Public Health,
Greater Glasgow Health Board, Glasgow

Preface

Whatever direction public health nursing in the UK will take, one issue underpins this nursing movement. Nurses need more information and specific training in order to fulfil their public health potential. It is intended that this book will act as an accessible introduction to many of the topic areas that underpin public health of particular relevance to nursing. Practical examples of nurses using public health approaches in their work are given to illustrate some nursing interpretations of public health activity.

In Section 1, some basic tools of public health are introduced. Epidemiology, health economics, commissioning, the social model of health and the potential for integrating public health and primary care are all presented with a nursing slant. Definitions of each discipline are combined with discussions of their relevance to nursing and examples and case studies are presented to bring the theoretical perspectives to life.

Section 2 covers some specific public health nursing interventions including needs assessment, population-based health promotion strategies, community development, communicable diseases and screening. Again, contemporary practice in these fields is described and discussed.

Finally, Section 3 examines some policy issues for nursing in relation to public health by looking at nurses' contributions to health information systems, measuring health outcomes and a discussion of the policy implications of population-based care for nurses.

1

The nursing contribution to public health

Pauline Craig

INTRODUCTION

Much has been written in recent years about the contribution of nurses in the UK to public health (e.g. RCN 1994, SNMAC 1995). There are as yet no clear definitions of nurses' public health roles in the UK, although there is some evidence that public health nursing has never been defined adequately in any country. A debate has been stimulated in the UK that has ranged from individual attempts to clarify nurses' public health roles (e.g. Billingham 1994a) to grim caveats about the potential for public health nursing to fulfil only bureaucratic functions within the NHS (Caraher & McNab 1996).

In the UK some of the confusion over public health nursing may be reflecting the lack of a clear definition of public health. For example, Lewis (1991) states that while the current definition of public health medicine emphasises health promotion and ill health prevention, NHS public health departments focus on the analysis of health service needs. Similarly, while UK nursing bodies produced documents about community nurses' public health functions, primary care reforms during the 1990s continued to draw nurses into more individualised, medical models of practice.

In examining the relationship between nurses and public health, it is impossible to avoid the term 'public health nursing'. Since creeping into nursing terminology in the UK in the 1990s, it has been used to describe the general contribution to public health of all nursing but also in relation to some diverse nursing specialities, for example infection control nursing and community-focused health visiting. In addition, there has been little discussion of the relationship between public health nursing in the UK and public health nursing in other countries, where the term has been used for much longer.

1

This chapter explores some of the definitions of public health nursing. It outlines the confusion around the term, identifies the roots of public health nursing within and outside the UK and provides an international perspective on contemporary public health nursing. In order to explain the potential relationship between nursing and public health, nursing is set into context with current public health practice, the new public health movement and Health for All.

ROOTS OF PUBLIC HEALTH NURSING IN THE US AND UK

Lillian Wald, the American nursing visionary, is said to have coined the term 'public health nursing' in the 1890s. She used her experiences in caring for the sick poor in the New York slums to convince policy makers about the social, economic and environmental causes of ill health she encountered (Frachel 1988). The early public health nurses developed a wide-ranging role, encompassing the following.

- They used a combination of epidemiology and 'womanly qualities'
- They worked with families living in poverty
- Advocacy
- Campaigning
- Health education
- Sick nursing (Frachel 1988)

Public health nursing in the United States was therefore founded on the recognition of poverty and the need for public services to be responsive to diverse socioeconomic and cultural groups (Erickson 1996).

A contemporary model of public health nursing in the United States has been described by Kuss et al (1997) who identified a number of concepts underlying public health nursing including:

- community empowerment;
- public health nursing history and nursing education;
- core public health functions, target populations and outcomes;
- environmental forces;
- caring;
- interdisciplinary collaboration;
- community partnership.

However, the development of public health nursing within primary care in the United States was hampered by the emphasis that health-care organisations placed on illness and role confusion with other nurses such as nurse practitioners (Laffrey & Page 1989).

Public health nursing exists in many countries and appears to have various forms. Khan & Landes (1993) found that, while underlying principles differed markedly from country to country, public health nurses in the UK, Finland, Sweden, Canada and the USA shared a number of common features.

- They focused on a defined community rather than individuals or families.
- There was an emphasis on disease prevention and health promotion as well as curative medicine.
- They performed an outreach function involving case finding and consultation.
- They had professional autonomy.

In their review, Khan & Landes (1993) identified only two public health nurses in the UK. They were both working in experimental pilot projects outwith mainstream community nursing, using community development approaches to assessing needs and working with the community to meet those needs (Khan & Landes 1993). In the United States, a community development approach is also taken by public health nurses. Examples of evaluated public health nurse programmes described by Deal (1994) included working with volunteers in a pregnancy and antenatal outreach programme and collaborating with communities to promote city-wide clean air policies.

Despite some common threads, public health activities of nurses in the UK evolved in a different way from those in the United States. Public health nursing in the US grew directly from nursing which was organised by voluntary associations outside medical supervision, resulting in autonomous practice (Frachel 1988). The early American nursing leaders were ambivalent about the increasing authority of medicine and were more influenced by the progressive politics of the feminist movement and social reform (Boschma 1997).

In contrast, health visiting in the UK appears to have developed in line with the dominance of male and medical dogma. In the 19th century, domiciliary nurses in the UK were mostly trained and organised by religious societies (Webster 1993). Health visiting developed in a separate process from home nursing services and became established as part of the UK public health movement of the late 19th century (Dingwall 1977). The roots of health visiting are believed to lie in both sanitary inspection, where male sanitary inspectors objected to women taking on their work, and addressing infant mortality, with medical officers of health (MOH) supporting the notion of the health visitor as 'mother's friend' (Davies 1988). As part of the public health establishment, health visiting was accountable to MOHs until 1974 and was not exclusively a nursing speciality until 1962 (Robinson 1982).

The early health visitors shared some of the concerns of the first American public health nurses: for example, recognition of the need to address social and environmental factors in improving health. Where their underlying principles differed was that health visiting in the UK was targeted by

MOHs at educating mothers in order to reduce infant mortality (Lewis 1991), whereas US public health nurses targeted communities in order to improve community health (Frachel 1988).

PUBLIC HEALTH NURSING VERSUS COMMUNITY HEALTH NURSING

The lack of consensus across different countries in the use of terms describing nurses working in the community may have contributed to the confusion over nurses' public health roles in some countries. The term 'community health nursing' is usually used as an umbrella term in the United States to describe all nurses working outside health institutions, including public health nurses (Scruby & McKay 1991). The main distinction between public health nurses and other community health nurses appears to be that in general, public health nurses focus on populations or communities whereas community health nurses target their services towards individuals and families (Deal 1994). However, that distinction can become blurred. For example, some public health nurses include direct nursing care within their broad remit of health promotion, community analysis and development (Laffrey & Page 1989). In addition, it appears that US public health nurses' target groups may differ depending on levels of qualification and experience, as Baccalaureate public health nurses focus on individuals and families and only at Masters or doctoral level do they focus on health needs of the community (Laffrey & Page 1989).

In parts of Canada, the terms 'public health nursing' and 'community health nursing' are also confused (King et al 1995). For example, a public health nursing service based in public health departments was first used in Alberta in 1918 to provide health education for schoolchildren and families. The term 'community health nursing' was introduced in the 1970s when the public health nursing service expanded to cover nursing the sick and disabled in the community, ironically very similar to Lillian Wald's public health nursing of the late 19th century. The terms are now used inconsistently in Canada, prompting King et al (1995) to recommend that 'public health nursing' be used to describe population-focused activities in health promotion and prevention of illness and accidents and 'community health nursing' as an umbrella term to include home health nursing, public health nursing and occupational nursing.

While 'community health nursing' is used as an umbrella term in some countries, 'public health nursing' appears to be the umbrella term used in Ireland to describe all nurses working in the community. The current Irish public health nursing service was set up in 1956 as an amalgamation of local authority nurses concerned with public health and the voluntary district nursing service (Hanafin 1997). In general, Irish public health nurses focus on individualised care and health promotion, mostly with children and elderly people, although they work in geographical areas and have a mandate to include work at the community level (McDonald & Chavasse 1997). Despite this community mandate, McDonald & Chavasse (1997) found a lack of management support, as well as a lack of confidence in practitioners, for the public health nurses' role in developing community participation.

MODERN PUBLIC HEALTH NURSING IN THE UK

The term 'public health nursing' is relatively new to the UK (Khan & Landes 1993). It appears to have been introduced early in the 1990s without proper definition and has sparked off wide debate and some confusion about the potential roles of nurses in relation to public health. The Standing Nursing and Midwifery Advisory Committee (SNMAC) (1995) stated that all nurses, midwives and health visitors have a contribution to make to public health but also picked out health visitors as 'public health workers in the entirety of their role'. The RCN (1994) outlined the issues for nurses taking on public health activity but did not specify which nurses and under which circumstances they might be able to fulfil a public health function. In addition, health visitors, district nurses, midwives and practice nurses have been described as 'all nurses working within public health' (Smith 1997), while Caraher & McNab (1996) suggest that the 'so-called' public health nursing posts that do exist in the UK may be no more than extended health visitor or district nurse roles.

Adding to the confusion is the lack of agreement on naming the population-focused activity. For example, a study of 29 health visitors with community-focused remits identified 13 different job titles for very similar remits, including: health visitor, public health nurse, public health health visitor, community development health visitor, community health development worker and community health worker (Craig 1998). There are therefore many ways in which to interpret 'public health nursing' in the UK and the muddle is far from being resolved.

Nursing and public health departments

Looking to public health theory and practice may be one way of identifying the relationship between nursing and public health. Since the NHS and Community Care Act of 1990, NHS public health departments focus on the analysis of health service needs (Lewis 1991). Responsibilities of public health doctors include ensuring that the medical profession and other healthcare professionals, health authorities, scientists and politicians are working towards improving the public health (Bhopal 1993). The definition of public health that underpins current public health practice is 'the science and art of preventing disease, prolonging life and promoting health through organised efforts of society' (DoH 1988). This definition is based on the WHO broad definition of health and consistent with the Ottawa Charter for Health Promotion and the Health for All policies (SNMAC 1995).

If public health practice is mostly about needs analysis and facilitating other professionals in improving health, there is no clear role here for nurses. Nurses are scarce in senior positions within commissioning and purchasing (SNMAC 1995) and there are no established career pathways for nurses to increase their numbers at decision-making levels (Salvage 1993). The other possibility for establishing the relationship between nurses and public health would be to examine the WHO principles underlying the 1988 definition of public health in order to explore a theoretical link.

Nursing and HFA

The Health for All by the Year 2000 (HFA) movement began in 1977 when the WHO adopted a resolution for citizens to attain a level of health by the year 2000 that will allow a socially and economically productive life (Salvage 1993). In 1981, a global strategy was adopted by many governments who produced local targets for achieving the goal of HFA (Salvage 1993). HFA also acted as a springboard for developing the concept of health promotion (Ashton & Seymour 1988). In 1986 the Ottawa Charter for Health Promotion was adopted, in which health promotion is based on five principles as follows.

1. Build public policies which support health.
2. Create supportive environments.
3. Strengthen community action – community development.
4. Develop personal skills to take control over health and environment.
5. Reorientate health services so that individuals, communities, health professionals and governments can work together towards a health-care system that contributes to 'health' (Ashton & Seymour 1988).

The Ottawa Charter provided the basis for the WHO Healthy Cities Project which was set up to develop processes to enable people in cities to live healthier lives (Curtice 1993). For example, the Glasgow Healthy City Project set up partnerships between the two local authorities and the health board to develop an integrated City Health Plan, addressing the social and economic conditions affecting health (Glasgow Healthy City Project 1995). Another aspect of the Glasgow Healthy City Project was to set up a network of community health projects, three of which had health visitor involvement (Craig 1995).

The WHO also defined a role in HFA for all nurses, midwives and health visitors in Europe (Salvage 1993). The key concept of this was to create a nursing role that is responsive to people's health needs rather than to the needs of the health-care system. The principles of the HFA nurse were said to be in line with the European policies of HFA and primary care, as follows.

- Positive health promotion
- Participation of individuals, families and communities in care

- Working towards equity
- Collaborative working
- Assurance of quality of care

It was recommended that education, management and planning of nursing services should take account of HFA principles and that nurses should be more involved in debating health policy (Salvage 1993).

Despite this vision of nursing, it could be argued that nurses' activity explicitly addressing issues that underpin HFA has been marginalised from core nursing services. For example, it has been observed that nurses taking community empowerment approaches remain outside mainstream services, such as health visitors working with families in poverty (Blackburn 1996), in community health projects (Craig 1998) and Irish public health nurses focusing on community participation (McDonald & Chavasse 1997). In addition, nursing is absent from discussions on the European Healthy Cities Project (e.g. Davies & Kelly 1993, Curtice 1993).

HEALTH VISITORS AS PUBLIC HEALTH NURSES

While all nurses have a potential public health role (SNMAC 1995), it appears that health visiting in particular has attracted the title 'public health nurse'. For example, the SNMAC (1995) claimed that health visiting was all about public health because of its role in health promotion with individuals and communities. However, this is misleading for two reasons. First, public health in health visiting is variously interpreted as activity relating to public health medicine priorities, for example contact tracing for TB (Chapter 9) or health service needs assessment (Chapter 7), but the term is also used to describe health visitors carrying out community development activity (Chapter 8). Second, health visitors are unlikely to be able to carry out community-focused health promotion activity when they are attached to GP practices. Any community-based health visiting activity tends to take place outwith mainstream primary care activity (Chapter 11).

Before jumping too quickly to the conclusion that health visiting is a good resting place for the public health title, there is a need to examine the implications for health visiting policy and practice. From the literature, it could be concluded that there are two angles from which to view the contemporary relationship between health visiting and public health: either health visiting is one of the many disciplines that contribute to public health or public health activity is one aspect of health visiting.

Health visiting as a branch of public health

This view is akin to the 'traditional' understanding of the function of health visiting, despite health visitors not having been attached to departments of public health since the 1970s. Contemporary NHS public health departments do not appear to recognise health visiting as a public health function and health visitors' public health activities, however they are defined, are generally developed outwith public health departments. Simultaneously, the current direction of primary care structures is drawing health visitors further into primary care, resulting increasingly in the need to work with a medical individualistic approach and less with a population focus (Symonds 1997).

Public health as a branch of health visiting

Alternatively, public health as one aspect of health visiting might refer to health visitors who work with a collective approach, focusing on population or community health needs rather than individual ones (Billingham 1994a). Health visitor-led community health promotion initiatives have become more visible in recent years (Cowley 1996). Working closely with communities, some health visitors have adopted community development methods of working, emphasising a holistic approach and the importance of personal and community empowerment in improving health and well-being.

Most of the health visitors adopting a community development approach work in areas with multiple health and social needs, addressing issues of health inequalities and poverty (Craig & Smith 1998). Poverty is now recognised as a major public health problem and, as one in three children in the UK (1994 figures) is born into a family who qualifies for social fund payments (Laughlin & Black 1995), few health visitors can ignore poverty and health issues.

Blackburn (1991) identified that health visitors can take action with regard to families living in poverty with three broad types of response:

- profiling and monitoring to gather information which can be used for planning and working for social change;
- prevention and alleviation for families coping with the material and health effects of poverty;
- social change – directly challenging team, local and national policies.

Health-visiting responses to families in poverty are comparable to Whitehead's (1995) findings regarding policy responses to inequalities in health. Effective policies were found to act at one of the following four levels: strengthening individuals; strengthening communities; improving access to essential facilities and services; and encouraging macroeconomic and cultural change, with the most powerful focus for change being at level four (Whitehead 1995).

Examples can be demonstrated of health-visiting developments acting at each of the four policy levels.

Strengthening individuals

Sensitive and empowering responses are crucial, rather than the victim-blaming approach of traditional health education messages (Russell 1995).

Health visitors can work to increase material or personal resources, e.g. through helping to claim benefits (Billingham 1994b) or child safety equipment loan schemes (Boyd et al 1993), and through counselling and support or developing self-esteem and skills as in the Community Mothers Programme (Whitehead 1995).

Strengthening communities

Health visitor caseload information has been used to study the relationship between health and material deprivation as it was seen as more readily updated than census data and easier to identify the relationship between factors affecting health (Shephard 1996). In addition, collecting information at community level, for example through community profiling, is an important part of planning for community-focused interventions and is a routine health-visiting activity in some areas (Cernik & Wearne 1994). A community development approach is often used by health visitors in conjunction with communities to take action on issues raised through profiling.

Improving access to essential facilities and services

Advocacy at an individual or community level is one area often seen as a core health-visiting activity (Twinn & Cowley 1992), for example in pursuing adequate housing or social services. De La Cuesta (1994) identified the existence of 'fringe work' used by health visitors to tailor services to the needs of clients, stretching resources to overcome deficiencies in health and social services. Examples included providing food, clothes or money and setting up support groups (De La Cuesta 1994).

Encouraging macroeconomic and cultural change

The health-visiting principle of 'influencing policies affecting health'* relates directly to this level of intervention. Health visitors can and do challenge local and national policies that create and maintain family poverty. Activity could include supporting local health campaigns or raising awareness among local people and politicians of the links between poor housing and health. In addition, health visitors could lobby managers and decision makers within health services to address poverty and health issues (Blackburn 1991).

Consequently, the role of health visitors as public health nurses is broad and cannot easily be defined within a medical model. Alternatively, public

---

*There are four principles underpinning health visiting in the UK, developed in 1977 and still relevant today (Twinn & Cowley 1992). They are: searching for health needs; raising awareness of health needs; facilitating health-enhancing behaviour; and influencing policies affecting health.

health in health visiting can be viewed from the perspective of a social model of health (see Chapter 5 for full discussion of the social model).

Health visiting, nursing and the new public health

If a population perspective, the adoption of community development methods of working and recognition of health inequalities are the elements of public health health visiting, it may be that nursing and public health meet in the new public health movement. In 1974, a Canadian report recognised health as being a function of a combination of lifestyle and the environment as well as being influenced by human biology and health-care provision (Donaldson & Donaldson 1993). This marked the beginning of a new public health movement which combined environmental change, i.e. physical, socioeconomic and psychological circumstances, with personal preventive measures, eschewing a victim-blaming approach and recognising the importance of the social aspects of health problems which are under-pinned by issues of local and national public policy. The new public health movement was supported by the development of the HFA policies (Ashton & Seymour 1988).

As for nursing in general and HFA, there is little policy support for health visitors working with a community-empowering approach to addressing health inequalities. This 'new public health' role for health visitors would only be legitimised if there were policy support in place for public health departments to tackle inequality in health status as well as inequality in health services uptake and then only if public health departments recognised this potential for health visiting. At the time of writing, the public health Green Papers had been published and they suggested that policy support for this way of working may be possible. However, at this point in time, health visiting is more closely associated with primary care which does not provide for health visiting to work outwith an individualistic way with general practice patients.

CONCLUSION: WOULD THE REAL PUBLIC HEALTH NURSES PLEASE STAND?

It appears that if public health nursing is to develop as a legitimate force in the UK, there is much work to be done to establish a meaningful role. The SNMAC (1995) stated that all nurses, midwives and health visitors have a contribution to make to public health and gave the following examples, stating that the list is not exhaustive.

- Nurse adviser in a health authority, carrying out needs assessment, purchasing, commissioning.
- Health visitor undertaking public health work allied to primary care, assessing needs at community level, client education, empowerment, collaboration.

- Specialist health visitor for health and homelessness in a deprived inner city.
- Staff nurse in intensive care carrying out accident prevention education in schools.
- Infection control nurse working with a consultant in communicable disease control.
- Community infection control nurse employed by a community health trust.

It is clear that there is no one branch of nursing that can claim the public health title. If nurses want to colonise NHS public health departments, there will need to be greater support for nurses to increase their numbers at the needs analysis and decision-making levels. On the other hand, if the public health role is to work with and advocate for communities, there must be policy support for nurses to work with a population focus and for targeting health inequalities. Boschma (1997) stated that competing views of public health nurse roles hindered the development of an infrastructure for early American public health nurses. Nurses in the UK need to prevent the debate strangling the further development of public health nursing. As nurses, we must establish our own potential for improving public health in order to move the public health agenda forward.

REFERENCES

Ashton J, Seymour H 1988 The new public health. Open University Press, Milton Keynes
Bhopal R S 1993 Public health medicine and purchasing health care. British Medical Journal 306: 381–382
Billingham K 1994a Beyond the individual. Health Visitor 67(9): 295
Billingham K 1994b The challenge for practice. Nursing Times 90(39): 43
Blackburn C 1991 Family poverty: what can health visitors do? Health Visitor 64(1): 368–370
Blackburn C 1996 Poverty perspective in health visiting practice. In: Bywaters P, McLeod E (eds) Working for equality in health. Routledge, London
Boschma G 1997 Ambivalence about nursing's expertise: the role of a gendered holistic ideology in nursing, 1890–1990. In: Rafferty AM, Robinson J, Elkan R (eds) Nursing history and the politics of welfare. Routledge, London
Boyd M, Brummell K, Billingham K, Perkins E 1993 The public health post at Strelley: an interim report. Nottingham Community Health NHS Trust, Nottingham
Caraher M, McNab M 1996 The public health nursing role: an overview of future trends. Nursing Standard 10(51): 44–48
Cernik K, Wearne M 1994 Promoting the integration of primary care and public health. Nursing Times 90(43): 44–45
Cowley S 1996 Reflecting on the past; preparing for the next century. Health Visitor 69(8): 313–316
Craig P 1995 A different role: health visiting in a community health project. Glasgow Healthy City Project, Glasgow
Craig P 1998 A description of the public health role of health visitors. Unpublished MSc thesis, University of Glasgow
Craig P, Smith L 1998 Health visiting and public health: back to our roots or a new branch? Health and Social Care in the Community 6(3): 172–180
Curtice L 1993 Strategies and values: research and the WHO Healthy Cities Project in Europe. In: Davies J K, Kelly M (eds) Healthy Cities: research and practice. Routledge, London
Davies C 1988 The health visitor as mother's friend: a woman's place in public health 1900–14. Social History of Medicine 1(1): 39–59

Davies J K, Kelly M (eds) 1993 Healthy cities research and practice. Routledge, London

De La Cuesta C 1994 Marketing: a process in health visiting. Journal of Advanced Nursing 19: 347–353

Deal L W 1994 The effectiveness of community nursing interventions: a literature review. Public Health Nursing 11(5): 315–323

Department of Health 1988 Public health in England: the report of the Committee of Inquiry into the Future Development of the Public Health Function. HMSO, London

Dingwall R 1977 Collectivism, regionalism and feminism: health visiting and British social policy 1850–1975. Journal of Social Policy 6(3): 291–315

Donaldson R J, Donaldson L J 1993 Essential public health medicine. Kluwer Academic Publishers, Lancaster

Erickson G P 1996 To pauperize or empower: public health nursing at the turn of the 20th and 21st centuries. Public Health Nursing 13(3): 163–169

Frachel R R 1988 A new profession: the evolution of public health nursing. Public Health Nursing 5(2): 86–90

Glasgow Healthy City Project 1995 Working Together for Glasgow's Health: Glasgow City Health Plan. Glasgow Healthy City Project, Glasgow

Hanafin S 1997 The role of the Irish public health nurse: manager, clinician and health promoter. Health Visitor 70(8): 295–297

Khan M, Landes R 1993 The role of the public health nurse – a review of the international literature. Public Health Research and Resource Centre, Salford

King M E, Harrison M J, Reutter L 1995 Public health nursing or community health nursing: examining the debate. Canadian Journal of Public Health 86(1): 24–25

Kuss T, Proulx-Girouard L, Lovitt S, Katz C B, Kenelly P 1997 A public health nursing model. Public Health Nursing 14(2): 81–91

Laffrey S C, Page G 1989 Primary health care in public health nursing. Journal of Advanced Nursing 14: 1044–1050

Laughlin S, Black D (eds) 1995 Poverty and health: tools for change. Public Health Alliance, Birmingham

Lewis J 1991 The public's health: philosophy and practice in Britain in the twentieth century. In: Fee E, Acheson R (eds) A history of education in public health. Oxford University Press, New York

McDonald A, Chavasse J 1997 Community participation within an Irish Health Board area. British Journal of Nursing 6(6): 341–345

RCN 1994 Public health: nursing rises to the challenge. Royal College of Nursing, London

Robinson J 1982 An evaluation of health visiting. Council for the Education and Training of Health Visitors, London

Russell J 1995 A review of health promotion in primary care. Greater London Association of Community Health Councils, London

Salvage J (ed) 1993 Nursing in action: strengthening nursing and midwifery to support Health For All. World Health Organisation, Copenhagen

Scruby L S, McKay M 1991 Strengthening communities: changing roles for community health nurses. Health Promotion International 6(4): 263–268

Shephard M 1996 Poverty, health and health visitors. Health Visitor 69(4): 141–143

Smith C 1997 Public health measurement. Nursing Management (UK) 3(9): 12–13

SNMAC 1995 Making it happen. Department of Health, London

Symonds A 1997 Ties that bind: problems with GP attachment. Health Visitor 70(2): 53–55

Twinn S, Cowley S 1992 The principles of health visiting: a re-examination. HVA and UKSC, London

Webster C (ed) 1993 Caring for health: history and diversity. Open University Press, Buckingham

Whitehead M (1995) Tackling inequalities: a review of policy initiatives. In: Benzeval M, Judge K, Whitehead M (eds) Tackling inequalities in health: an agenda for action. King's Fund, London

Core elements of public health

2

Applications of epidemiology in planning for health

Robert West

INTRODUCTION

Epidemiology is the core discipline of public health. The Greek origin of the word means simply the study of the people but during the 20th century it has taken on a more medical meaning so that now it encompasses the study of the distribution of disease in populations. It is easy, then, to see how this relates to the study of the health of populations or public health. The study of the distribution of disease in populations starts with observation and description of variations in the three dimensions of place, time and person. While epidemiology is generally thought of as a relatively recent medical discipline, the subject has very early antecedents. No student of public health should overlook the classic description by Hippocrates (1938) in *On airs, waters and places*.

Whoever wishes to investigate medicine properly should proceed thus: in the first place to consider the seasons of the year, and what effects each of them produces. Then the winds, the hot and the cold, especially such as are common to all countries, and then such as are peculiar to each locality. In the same manner, when one comes into a city to which he is a stranger, he should consider its situation, how it lies as to the winds and the rising of the sun; for its influence is not the same whether it lies to the north or the south, to the rising or to the setting sun. One should consider most attentively the waters which the inhabitants use, whether they be marshy and soft, or hard and running from elevated and rocky situations, and then if saltish and unfit for cooking; and the ground, whether it be naked and deficient in water, or wooded and well watered, and whether it lies in a hollow, confined situation, or is elevated and cold; and the mode in which the inhabitants live, and what are their pursuits, whether they are fond of drinking and eating to excess, and given to indolence, or are fond of exercise and labour.

This encapsulated the principles of epidemiological enquiry over 2000 years ago and summarises with disarming clarity several important determinants of health (or illness), many of which are still relevant today.

Study of disease variations in place, time and person has two main objectives: first, by description of numbers with the disease, to assist planners in assessment of need, and second, by examination of association with environmental or temporal factors or personal characteristics, to assist clinicians in explaining aetiology. This latter objective has been for many years the principal focus of most epidemiologists and pursuit of this objective has given rise to most developments in epidemiological methods. The main reason for the concentration on this area probably lies with the primacy of diagnosis as the intellectual challenge of clinical medicine. From a public health perspective, good epidemiological studies that lead to identification of likely cause, or at least likely partial cause in diseases with multifactorial aetiology, certainly offer the greatest opportunities for prevention. In a brief introduction to epidemiology and its applications to public health, there is a logic in expanding first on 'needs assessment' and health-care planning, the reason being that 'needs assessment' mostly involves counting the numbers of people in need.

MEASURING DISEASE FREQUENCY

The two measures of disease frequency are *incidence*, the number of new cases per unit time (per unit population), and *prevalence*, the number of existing cases (per unit population) (Last 1988). The former is used in acute disease, when the impact of the disease is its occurrence, like outbreaks of food poisoning, heart attacks or accidents. The latter is used to measure the burden of chronic disease, as for example in congenital anomalies, osteoarthritis or stroke.

It is important to establish a sound definition of disease before starting to count to estimate incidence or prevalence; even with international agreements on classification of disease, it is surprising what proportion of inter-regional or intercountry differences in apparent disease frequency can be attributed to differences in what counts as disease. A series of cross-sectional studies of the population to estimate incidence and prevalence of the relevant diseases should provide a picture of variation by place in, for example, pneumoconiosis (mostly attributable to coal dust), variation in time in, for example, the historic decline in tuberculosis or the seasonality of influenza and variation between individuals in, for example, lung cancer.

In the practical world of public health, it can be argued that 'needs assessment' implies a potential to treat, cure or care for those in need. There have been semantic debates on the taxonomy of need, for example 'absolute need' and 'addressable need', as well as consideration of the more practical 'met need' (those individuals who are counted in health services statistics) and 'unmet need', both those on the waiting list and those for whom there is no service (although the knowledge and technology may exist).

MORBIDITY AND MORTALITY STATISTICS

The burden of disease (incidence or prevalence) in a planning area is usually reported as mortality and morbidity statistics. Mortality often carries the most influence as the 'hard' statistic, although it has little relevance in many non-life threatening diseases or chronic diseases. Most countries publish mortality statistics, registered in protocols agreed with the World Health Organisation; in the UK this is done by the Office for National Statistics (ONS 1998). There are several points to note about mortality statistics: first, they are 'incidence' measures (people only die once). Second, while there may be little ambiguity about death (in most cases), there can be many differences over attributing the leading cause; for example, is breast cancer the cause or an accompanying condition? There are internationally agreed rules for the classification of cause of death (WHO 1992) but it has to be remembered that cause is ascribed by many doctors, most of whom are not thinking about public health statistics when they certify death. This links also to the third point about mortality data, that they are 'routine' rather than 'research' statistics. It follows, then, that a thorough (research) analysis of mortality might involve independent reclassification of underlying cause and independent reassessment of laboratory and autopsy reports.

Morbidity statistics are measures of illness, like the number of new heart attacks in a year (incidence), or incapacity, like the number with chronic osteoarthritis of the hip (prevalence), and are only truly measured by cross-sectional or repeated cross-sectional studies, for example the WHO MONICA project for heart disease (WHO 1989). It is a common misconception that morbidity is measured in health service use statistics but these latter are measures of 'met' need (see above). For some diseases 'met' need may be a fairly high proportion of the total number with disease and hence a useful proxy measure. For chronic diseases like cancer the registers are more reliable than health service use data like hospital discharge statistics, since procedures have been established to both seek registration from several sources and minimise double counting (OPCS 1994). Many communicable diseases are 'notifiable' and the regular reports of the communicable diseases surveillance centres (CDSC) (OPCS 1995) provide useful indicators of disease variation, but it should be recognised that notification rates in some of the notifiable diseases can be very low.

These routine health statistics, from hospitals, laboratories or general practice, etc., may provide useful information on patterns and trends. However, routine health service use and notification data should be interpreted with caution in assessment of need in health-care planning. Variations in place, time and person can all arise from artifacts. Studies have shown examples where these data are more closely related to health service provision than to incidence or prevalence of disease; *reductio ad absurdum*, if there is no facility to treat then there is no service utilisation (Baldwin et al 1987). A further consideration in needs assessment is whether or not there is a service that meets the need, a treatment that cures or improves prognosis or relieves pain and suffering. It can be argued that, if there is no treatment that works, need cannot be met and hence there would be little point in measuring such untreatable need. This will be discussed later.

AETIOLOGY

The study of variation in place, time and person to investigate aetiology or cause has been the favoured application of epidemiologists for many years. The design of observational studies to examine association between disease frequency and some environmental factor or personal habit or characteristic and the interpretation of such studies have provided most of the intellectual challenges for epidemiologists, rather as diagnosis has challenged clinicians. From the public health perspective, the objective of these studies of association is to identify cause so that the cause may be eliminated (if that is feasible) as, for example, in an outbreak of food poisoning or a contaminated water supply, or so that a contributory cause may be addressed as, for example, in cigarette smoking and heart disease.

The simplest type of epidemiological study to examine association, the case history study, is well illustrated by the example of scrotal cancer described by Percival Pott in 1775: a high proportion of young men with scrotal cancer were chimney sweeps and since the majority of young men were not chimney sweeps, it could be inferred that an exposure incurred in sweeping chimneys in the 18th century (and possibly to a lesser degree today) was associated with the disease. In this example the relative frequency of disease occurrence was so marked that a formal comparison with the non-diseased (controls) was unnecessary.

Nonetheless, this is a good introduction to the case control study, which estimates the exposure to a putative hazard (for example, soot) in 'cases', those with the disease under study (scrotal cancer), and 'controls', those without the disease (preferably healthy normal people). The case control study is the most widely used epidemiological method to investigate association, largely because it can be undertaken retrospectively and relatively quickly. When association is strong, as for example in cigarette smoking and lung cancer or salmonella in one dish of a buffet meal and gastrointestinal illness, the simple case control design may identify the putative hazard without difficulty. Problems arise in the study of many diseases of multifactorial origin; in many chronic diseases the relative risk associated with exposure to one contributory hazard may be 2 or less (for example, exposure to X-rays in utero and subsequent cancer in childhood). When a disease under study may have multifactorial aetiology and relative risk of any one putative hazard may not be high, great care is needed in selection of suitable 'controls' and in matching of controls to cases, on factors already known to be associated, and in treatment of potentially confounding variables (variables that may be associated with both exposure and outcome). Largely because of these potential difficulties, the greatest methodological

---

Case study 2.1 An example of a case control study: occupational and environmental exposure in patients with myelodysplastic syndromes

Background Previous studies had shown association between radiation and leukaemia; for example, fetal radiation and childhood leukaemia (Stewart et al 1958). Little was known of the aetiology of this relatively recently defined condition, the myelodysplastic syndromes (MDS or 'preleukaemia').
Cases 400 men and women with recently diagnosed MDS.
Controls 400 matched on sex, age within ±3 years and area of residence (health district, population ~ 100 000).
Occupational history Detailed questionnaire regarding exposure to list of 90 putative hazards including, e.g., benzene, herbicides and radiation.

Reported history of exposure to radiation	MDS patients ($n = 400$)	Controls (without MDS) ($n = 400$)
Yes	41	21
No	359	379

Thus, odds ratio = 2.1 (95% confidence interval 1.2–3.7). This means that MDS patients were rather more than twice as likely as sex, age and area of residence matched controls to report a history of exposure to radiation (source West et al 1995).

---

advances in epidemiology in the past 30 years have been seen in the design, analysis and interpretation of case control studies.

The alternative approach to study of association, the cohort study, is perhaps preferable in design. This is a prospective study of a group of people, some of whom may be exposed to the suspected hazard (or have the personal characteristic or habit) and some of whom may not, and comparison of the disease frequency among those exposed and not exposed. It has the advantages over the case control study that exposures may be measured (rather than 'recalled') and that disease incidence may be observed but it has the obvious disadvantages that many normal individuals may need to be measured and followed for many years to yield a meaningful number with disease. The matching and potential confounder problems of the case control study are lessened but not eliminated; for example, for several years after cohort studies showed an association between cigarette smoking and lung cancer, some eminent scientists argued the constitutional hypothesis – that a genetic factor predisposed towards both smoking and cancer.

Observational epidemiology yields association and cause can only truly be shown by experiment. Associations may arise by chance (statistical), through another factor (confounder), as a consequence or as a cause. Two useful criteria have been propounded to help in the interpretation of causality, explaining association in observational studies at two very different stages in the development of epidemiology. The Koch postulates

---

Case study 2.2   An example of a cohort study. Caerphilly heart disease study

Background   Previous studies like Framingham (Dawber 1980) have shown blood pressure, (total) blood cholesterol and smoking to be primary risk factors for ischaemic heart disease.

Design   A cohort of 4860 middle-aged men in Caerphilly (South Wales) and Speedwell (Bristol) recruited to study, interviewed (e.g. for diet), clinical examination (e.g. for prevalent heart disease) and measured (e.g. for anthropometric characteristics and blood chemistry). Individuals reinterviewed and reexamined periodically to ascertain incident (new) heart disease. After an average of 4 years, 251 men died of or experienced non-fatal myocardial infarction.

Fibrinogen (g/l)	Men at risk	New heart disease (fatal or non-fatal)	Relative risk*
<3.0	921	21	1.0
3.0–3.5	921	33	1.6
3.5–3.9	921	42	2.1
3.9–4.4	921	46	2.2
>4.4	921	89	4.1

*Adjusted for age. The relationship between fibrinogen and heart disease remains when adjusted for age, area, smoking, prevalent heart disease, blood pressure, body mass index and cholesterol. This study showed that fibrinogen is an independent 'risk factor' for heart disease (source Yarnell et al 1991).

---

were proposed to identify responsible organisms in the era of communicable disease epidemiology (Koch 1890) and the Bradford Hill criteria nearly a hundred years later were designed to assist interpretation of contributory causes in multifactorial disease aetiology in the era of chronic disease epidemiology (Bradford Hill 1965).

PUBLIC HEALTH PROGRAMMES

When research has satisfactorily identified likely cause or contributory cause, public health practitioners can design programmes with the objective of removing hazards or reducing exposures or educating the public about the risks attributed to certain habits and practices. In prevention, it is convenient to distinguish again between communicable and chronic disease. A typical outbreak investigation (of a communicable disease) follows an enquiry comparable to the research study, the principal difference being that the nature of the organism is known (once typed in the laboratory) and from past experience the likely source can be anticipated, which can lead to the source being identified quite rapidly. Once the source is identified and confirmed (using Koch's principles) legislation may facilitate removal of the contamination. The public health intervention over a (contributory) causal factor in chronic disease is rather different: since, for example, the role of cigarette smoking in lung cancer is well established, there is no need to seek the brand of cigarette or the source of cigarettes getting into the hands of teenagers.

The appropriate strategies for reducing exposure are education of individuals and public generally, legislation (on selling to the underaged and on advertising) and fiscal (raising the cost). In other chronic diseases, a contributory cause may be more amenable to removal (or removal for most people) even if the relative risks associated are quite modest, as for example in radiation and organic solvents and haematological malignancies. Many of the successful reductions in exposure during the second half of this century have been reductions in occupational exposure which, as we enter the 21st century, leaves public health with the problem of identifying lower levels of environmental exposure, as for example in landfill sites.

After 'true' prevention (removal) and 'attempted' prevention (legislation and education), mention should be made of screening, sometimes called 'secondary' prevention. Screening is again public health, since programmes are directed at populations rather than at sick individuals. In most examples, screening is early detection rather than true prevention. Useful criteria have been formulated by Wilson & Junger (1968) and others to assist public health practitioners in identifying diseases with suitable presymptomatic states, amenable to intervention that improves prognosis and appropriate tests that can detect the presymptomatic state with very high sensitivity and specificity (tests that may be useful in assisting diagnosis among the sick may not be good enough to employ on the outwardly healthy). It is interesting to observe that many of the screening activities currently being offered have not been evaluated against these criteria; indeed, one of the best known population-based screening programmes of the century, mass miniature X-ray for tuberculosis, never really satisfied all the criteria (pre-1950s there was no real treatment and post-1950s there were better screening tests).

Evaluation of screening programmes leads naturally to consideration of a final area of application of epidemiology in public health.

EFFECTIVENESS, EFFICACY AND EFFICIENCY

Health-care evaluation seeks to establish the efficacy, effectiveness and efficiency of health-care interventions and programmes of health-care intervention. Professional bodies have long sought to maintain standards but the inception of the NHS and the subsequent increasing demand on scarce resources and specialised technologies have focused the attention of many public health practitioners, particularly since the first of the NHS reorganisations in 1974. Cochrane (1973), the first president of the Faculty of Public Health Medicine (then Community Medicine), did much to focus attention on the three Es.

By efficacy we mean that the intervention (therapy) can work, that it is biologically possible in some laboratories, wards, hospitals, etc. Effectiveness means that, as a regular programme, it works on average, that the therapy gives a better prognosis or relieves pain better than placebo. Efficiency means that, as a regular programme, it gets a better result with use of fewer resources than some alternative. Efficiency is the lead into health economics (see Chapter 3).

Efficacy, effectiveness and efficiency all require defined objectives for treatment and outcome measures so that it can be seen that the objectives are achieved. The clearest evidence of effectiveness is that obtained by experiment, the randomised control trial. While trials are almost impractical and unusually unethical in aetiological study, their use in evaluating services has gained widespread acceptance since the MRC trial of streptomycin in tuberculosis (MRC 1950). However, although trials are regarded as the 'gold standard' in service evaluation and public health practice, there remain many instances when, in the prevailing state of knowledge, trials are unethical and/or impractical and it is necessary to draw inference from observational studies. These situations demand studies of the same rigorous design, analysis and interpretation as in aetiological studies. Thus, difference in outcome following surgery in different hospitals may be due to different technique, skill or competence but may be due to many other factors such as case mix, selection criteria and even choice of outcome measures while time trends in survival may be due to improving therapy or to changes in detection threshold (diagnosis and inclusion).

AUDIT

Finally, in ensuring that programmes achieve their objectives, there is a clear role for audit. When research has demonstrated programme effectiveness, audit ensures that the correct therapeutic programmes are followed. A couple of examples of the roles for observational study, randomised trials and service audit are aspirin for acute myocardial infarction (MI) and sleeping posture for sudden infant death syndrome (SIDS). In the former, the Boston Drug Surveillance Program observed that patients hospitalised for MI were less likely to have taken aspirin prior to admission than those admitted for other diagnosis (Boston Collaborative Drug Surveillance Group 1974). Randomised trials in Cardiff (Elwood et al 1974) and subsequently elsewhere showed that following MI, patients on aspirin were less likely to suffer further MI or death. There is now a role for clinical follow-up in outpatients, in rehabilitation programmes, by GPs or practice nurses to check that post-MI patients (and those deemed as at significant risk of MI) are taking aspirin regularly.

In the latter example, observational studies of SIDS identified posture as a possible contributory factor (among many others) to the unexplained deaths. The Back to Sleep campaign (an uncontrolled 'experiment') showed significant reduction in SIDS (DoH 1993) and there is now a role for health visitors checking that babies are the right way up (after an unfortunate decade of checking that babies were the wrong way up!).

CONCLUSION

In this chapter the definition of public health has been quite broad, in keeping with the Chief Medical Officer's recent working paper on 'improving the public health function' (CMO 1998). It is recognised that as many factors contribute to health, many agencies besides the NHS contribute or could contribute to public health. It is also appreciated that professionals from many disciplines, scattered through these many agencies, have roles to play in pursuit of public health. It follows that many professionals will benefit from a basic working appreciation of the principles of epidemiology.

In recent years we have seen a large increase in the number of Masters of Public Health courses, in the numbers of students attending these courses and in the variety of backgrounds from which these students are drawn. These developments are to be welcomed and can only strengthen the public health function and improve the public health.

REFERENCES

Baldwin J, Acheson E D, Graham W 1987 Textbook of medical record linkage. Oxford University Press, Oxford
Boston Collaborative Drug Surveillance Group 1974 Regular aspirin intake and acute myocardial infarction. British Medical Journal i: 440–443
Bradford Hill A 1965 The environment and disease, association or causation? Proceedings of the Royal Society of Medicine 58: 295–300
Chief Medical Officer 1998 Report to strengthen the public health function in England. Department of Health, London
Cochrane A L 1973 Effectiveness and efficiency. Nuffield Provincial Hospitals Trust, London
Dawber T R 1980 The Framingham study: epidemiology of atherosclerotic heart disease. Harvard University Press, Cambridge, MA
Department of Health 1993 Sleeping position of infants and cot death. Report of Chief Medical Officer. HMSO, London
Elwood P C, Cochrane A L, Burr M L et al 1974 A randomised controlled trial of acetyl salicylic acid in the secondary prevention of mortality from myocardial infarction. British Medical Journal i: 436–440
Hippocrates 1938 On airs, waters, and places. Translated and republished in Medical Classics 3: 19–42
Koch R 1890 Ueber bakteriologische Forschung. Verhandlungen X International Medicin Congress, Berlin
Last J M 1988 A dictionary of epidemiology. Oxford University Press, Oxford
Medical Research Council 1950 Clinical trials of antihistamine drugs in the prevention and treatment of the common cold. British Medical Journal ii: 425–429
Office for National Statistics 1998 Mortality statistics for England and Wales 1996. HMSO, London
OPCS 1994 Cancer statistics: registrations England and Wales 1989. HMSO, London

OPCS Communicable Disease Surveillance Centre 1995 Communicable disease statistics, England and Wales 1993. HMSO, London

Pott P 1775 Chirurgical observations relative to the cateract, the polypus of the nose, the cancer of the scrotum, the different kinds of rupture, and the mortification of the feet. Hawse, Clark and Collins, London

Stewart A, Webb J, Hewitt D 1958 A survey of childhood malignancies. British Medical Journal i: 1495–1508

West R R, Stafford D A, Farrow A, Jacobs A 1995 Occupational and environmental exposures and myelodysplasia: a case control study. Leukemia Research 19: 127–139

WHO 1989 WHO MONICA project: assessing CHD mortality and morbidity. International Journal of Epidemiology 1 (suppl): 520–527

WHO 1992 International classification of disease, 10th revision (ICD 10). World Health Organization, Geneva

Wilson J M G, Junger G 1968 Principles and practice of screening for disease. Public health papers. World Health Organisation, Geneva

Yarnell J W G, Bainton D, Sweetnam P M et al 1991 Fibrinogen, viscosity and white cell count are major risk factors for ischaemic heart disease: the Caerphilly and Speedwell Collaborative Heart Disease Studies. Circulation 83: 836–844

FURTHER READING

Abramson J H 1990 Survey methods in community medicine. Churchill Livingstone, Edinburgh

Black N, Boswell D, Gray A, Murphy S, Popay J 1984 Health and disease. Open University Press, Milton Keynes

Donaldson R J 1993 Essential public health medicine. Kluwer, Dordrecht

Farmer R, Miller D 1982 Epidemiology of diseases. Blackwell, Oxford

Frankel S J, West R R 1992 Rationing and rationality in the NHS: the persistence of writing lists. Macmillan, Basingstoke

Lilienfeld D E, Stolley P D 1994 Foundations of epidemiology, 3rd edn. Oxford University Press, Oxford

MacMahon B, Pugh T F 1970 Epidemiology principles and methods. Little, Brown, Boston

Meredith Davies B 1995 Public health, preventive medicine and social services. Baillière Tindall, London

Sackett D L, Haynes R B, Guyatt G H, Tugwell P 1991 Clinical Epidemiology. Little, Brown, Boston

Stevens A, Raffery J 1994 Health care needs assessment. Radcliffe Medical, Oxford

St Leger A S, Schnieden H, Walsworth-Bell J P 1992 Evaluating health services' effectiveness. Open University Press, Buckingham

3

Economic evalution

Mandy Ryan   Emma McIntosh

INTRODUCTION

This chapter looks at the contribution health economics can make to the efficient allocation of scarce health-care resources. Central to the discipline of economics are the concepts of 'scarcity', 'choice' and 'opportunity cost'. Each of these concepts is outlined in the following sections. Resources are 'scarce'; every time we 'choose' to use them in one way we give up the 'opportunity' of using them in other ways. Thus, the implication of scarcity, choice and opportunity cost is that priorities have to be set. Economic evaluation can be seen as a framework to assist in priority setting by analysing the costs and benefits of alternative health-care interventions. It is a decision-aiding instrument for the allocation of society's scarce health-care resources. This chapter outlines the various costs and benefits relevant to health-care and then describes how these costs and benefits are brought together in an evaluative framework.

In the next section issues arising in the identification and valuation of costs are considered. The reader will become familiar with important concepts in costing exercises, such as: opportunity cost; the margin; discounting; and sensitivity analysis. The main types of costs to be considered in an economic evaluation will then be summarised, with consideration given to how to identify and collect such data, taking account of the key concepts already introduced. Attention will then turn to benefit assessment. Two issues are discussed: what is it we are trying to measure and how can we measure such factors? It is argued that despite the emphasis on health outcomes in recent years, benefit assessment in health economics should also consider non-health outcomes and process attributes. Attention is then given to methods of valuing health outcomes, non-health outcomes and process attributes. Four benefit assessment tools are introduced: clinical measures of outcome; quality-adjusted life years (QALYs) (using visual analogue, standard gamble and time trade-off); willingness to pay (WTP); and conjoint analysis (CA). Following this, it is shown how costs and benefits can be brought together in a formal economic evaluation. Readers are introduced to cost-effectiveness analysis (CEA), cost-utility analysis (CUA) and cost-benefit analysis (CBA).

An important point to note is that not all possible costs and benefits have to be or indeed should be included within every economic evaluation. It depends upon the perspective of the evaluator as to which are the 'relevant' costs and benefits. A purchaser may only be interested in health service costs and benefits whilst an evaluation from the patient's perspective may only be concerned with patient costs and benefits, not those associated with the health service. A societal perspective would consider all costs and benefits to all sectors of society such as the provider, purchaser, clinician voluntary organisation, patient and friends.

ISSUES IN COSTINGS

Opportunity cost

The economic concept of cost is 'opportunity cost'. This concept takes as its starting point the premise that resources are scarce. Therefore, every time we choose to use resources in one way, we are giving up the 'opportunity' of using them in other beneficial activities. The opportunity cost of any health-care intervention is therefore defined as the benefit lost by *not* using that resource in its best alternative use. Only if a resource has a next best use does it have an opportunity cost. The concept of opportunity cost also embodies the crucial notion of sacrifice: in economics something only has 'value' if a sacrifice has been made or is being made for it.

Using this definition of cost, items to be included on the cost side of an economic evaluation are any 'resources' which have an alternative use. Often, costs (and benefits) are misclassified within economic evaluations (Donaldson & Shackley 1997). For example, anxiety has often been counted as a 'cost' and cost savings as 'benefits'. However, anxiety per se does not have an 'opportunity cost' – it is not a resource which could be used in some other activity. Anxiety is a negative effect on health or well-being and should be accounted for on the benefit side of an evaluation. Likewise, 'cost savings' are negative costs and should be accounted for on the cost side.

The importance of the margin

An important concept in costing (and benefit) exercises is that of the margin. The margin is concerned with change. The marginal cost is the cost/saving of producing one unit more/less of a programme. Decisions about the allocation of scarce health-care resources are usually concerned not with whether to introduce a service but rather whether to expand or reduce a service. For example, with regard to screening for cervical cancer, the question is usually whether the screening interval should be changed from 3 years to 1 year or the age for screening should be reduced rather than whether screening should be provided at all. Given this, costing studies should be mainly concerned with measuring marginal costs, not the generally more accessible but often inappropriate average costs.

The importance of distinguishing marginal costs from average costs was clearly demonstrated in the work of Neuhauser & Lewicki (1975), based on the American Cancer Society's protocol of six sequential stool tests to detect the presence of colonic cancer. Table 3.1 shows the results from this study. The average cost per case detected of the sixth test was estimated to be $2451. However, the marginal cost involved in detecting one extra case of cancer was $47 million. Whilst this study does not provide an answer to the question 'How many tests are worthwhile?', it demonstrates clearly the additional resources that would have to be spent to detect an extra case of colon cancer. It therefore provides policy makers with better information concerning the real opportunity cost of detecting an extra cancer case.

Jacobs & Baladi (1996) address the issue of bias in cost measurement. Such biases, they argue, reflect the divergence of 'cost' from the desired 'marginal cost' measure. The biases they identify are defined as: scale bias; case mix bias; methods bias; and site selection bias. *Scale bias* occurs when the department is operating at a point where the average cost does not equal the marginal cost but the evaluator makes the assumption that marginal cost equals average cost. *Case mix bias* occurs when the measure of quantity chosen is not accurate and so the unit cost for that service or case over- or

Table 3.1 The importance of the margin in costing – incremental cases detected and incremental, average and marginal costs ($) of sequential guaiac tests

Number of tests	Total number of cases detected	Incremental number of cases detected	Total cost[a]	Incremental cost	Average cost[b]	Marginal cost[c]
1	65.9469	65.946	77 511	77 511	1175	1175
2	71.4424	5.4956	107 690	30 179	1507	5492
3	71.9004	0.4580	130 199	22 509	1810	49 150
4	71.9385	0.0382	148 116	17 917	2059	469 534
5	71.9417	0.0032	163 141	15 024	2268	4 724 695
6	71.9420	0.0003	176 331	13 190	2451	47 107 214

[a] Calculated by addition of cost of guaiac stool testing on 10 000 people and cost of barium enema examination on all those with positive tests.
[b] Calculated by division of total costs by total no. of cases detected
[c] Calculated by division of incremental costs by incremental gain in cases detected

underestimates the actual amount of resources used; for example, when average patient days are used as a measure of quantity, cases which are resource intensive will have their costs understated. *Methods bias* occurs when the incorrect measurement technique is used; for example, if costs are fixed then bias is created if these costs are treated as variable. *Site selection bias* might occur where costs are measured at a single site. A cost which is taken at one site may misrepresent the marginal cost in the average site. This bias can be adjusted for if data on costs are collected for all relevant sites.

Discounting

Costs (and benefits) of health-care interventions can occur at different times. For example, in prevention programmes costs are incurred early in the scheme whereas the benefits may stretch years into the future. Individuals generally prefer to incur costs in the future (and receive benefits sooner). Given this preference, costs that are incurred in the future should be given less weight, i.e. be discounted. The greater the preference for costs to occur in the future, the higher the discount rate. Currently, the UK Treasury recommends a discount rate of 6%. Using this discount rate and the figures in Table 3.3 (p. 31), £1 spent in year 0 (i.e. those costs occurring now) is worth £1; £1 spent in year 1 is worth £0.94 pence (or has a weight of 0.94); £1 spent in year 2 is worth £0.89 pence (or has a weight of 0.89) and so on. It is clear to see that the further into the future costs occur, the less weight they are given. Table 3.2 shows the effects of discounting at 6%. Imagine a new type of operation is being introduced which is less costly at the outset but gives rise to a number of retreatments. Undiscounted, the new operation appears more expensive. However, it is only by discounting the future retreatments that the true costs are displayed which show the new operation to be less expensive.

Sensitivity analysis

Every evaluation will contain some degree of uncertainty, imprecision or methodological controversy and as a result assumptions will have to be made (Drummond et al 1987). What if disposable equipment was used

Table 3.2 The importance of discounting in costing

Alternatives	Year 0	Year 1	Year 2	Year 3	Total costs
Old operation	£2500	£0	£0	£0	£2500
New operation (undiscounted)	£1050	£500*	£500*	£500*	£2550
(discounted)	£1050	£471.70	£445	£419.80	£2386.50

*Adjusted for the effects of inflation

instead of reusable in laparoscopic surgery? What would be the effect on costs if length of stay was 3 days instead of 2? What if patient costs were included in the analysis? What if a discount rate of 3% was used instead of 6%? Sensitivity analysis allows the testing of the sensitivity of the results to the assumptions made. For a comprehensive summary of the main types of uncertainty and the corresponding role of sensitivity analysis in addressing this, see Briggs et al (1994).

Categorising resources to be included within economic evaluations

Box 3.1 provides guidance on costs to be included in an economic evaluation. Staffing costs often comprise the largest component of health-care resources, e.g. in an operating theatre the ratio of staff to patients may be as high as 7:1. There will only be an opportunity cost of staff time if time released could be used in an alternative way, i.e. patient care. This may be illustrated by thinking about the introduction of midwife-led antenatal care (Ratcliffe et al 1996). If any released obstetrician time is used to do something of equal value or savings are realised by the freeing-up of their time, then this cost saving can be valued at the obstetrician's market value, i.e. their salary plus on-costs (such as National Insurance and superannuation). However, the introduction of midwife-led care may not release staff time which can

---

Box 3.1   Guidance on costs to be included in an economic evaluation

Direct costs
Health-care resources
- Staffing
- Consumables, e.g. drugs
- Overheads, e.g. administration and laundry
- Capital, e.g. buildings and equipment

Related services
- Community services, e.g. community nurse specialising in the care of people with HIV/AIDS
- Ambulance services, e.g. for accident and emergency
- Voluntary services, e.g. voluntary workers in residential hostels for people with mental health problems

Costs to patients and their families/friends
- Extra expenses incurred through treatments, e.g. over-the-counter drugs or medical aids and adaptations
- Additional costs of being in hospital/at GP, e.g. childminding expenses
- Travel costs to and from GP/hospital
- Time lost from work

Indirect costs
- Time lost from work
- Costs external to health and welfare services

be used for activities that have an equal value. This is often dealt with by the use of sensitivity analysis, where assumptions have to be made concerning what proportion of the released staff time has an equivalent value (see below) and indeed if there is any alternative use of released resources (Ratcliffe et al 1996).

Consumables are items which are used for or on behalf of each patient such as drugs, dressings, disposable equipment and sutures. Consumables are replaced on a regular basis, hence monetary unit costs are usually an appropriate reflection of opportunity cost as well as being readily available.

Overhead costs are those costs shared by more than one programme, e.g. heat and light, laundry, cleaning and administration. These services are provided centrally and costs are apportioned amongst the various sectors using various means. The most favoured technique is marginal analysis. Here an attempt is made to see which costs, if any, would change if a given service or provision were introduced or removed from the overall activity. Thus, it may be concluded that overhead costs are zero for a proposed health-care intervention if such costs will not change as a service is changed, increased or decreased. An alternative, and possibly easier, technique for taking account of overhead costs is to calculate per diem or average costs, i.e. total operating costs divided by total patient utilisation. However, a limitation of this approach is that it is only valid for truly 'average' patients and therefore often does not reflect the true opportunity cost. For a description of the various methods of overhead allocation, see Drummond et al (1987).

Capital items include land and building as well as large items of equipment. Despite an initial outlay, the opportunity costs of capital are spread over time. This is accounted for by spreading the opportunity cost of capital assets over the number of years of life judged relevant. One way of doing this is to calculate an equivalent annual cost (EAC). Using this method, the initial outlay on a capital asset is converted to an annual sum which, when paid over the estimated lifespan of the equipment, would equal the resources invested plus their opportunity cost. This EAC takes account of the fact that the resources invested to purchase the capital equipment could have earned a certain rate of interest if invested, i.e. it takes account of their opportunity cost, the foregone benefits of its next best use. Equivalent annual costs are readily available (Table 3.3). If an item of surgical equipment cost £1000 and has a lifespan of 5 years, and assuming a discount rate of 6%, this would be 'equivalent' to five annual payments of £237.40. This higher total cost of £1187 (5 × £237.40) reflects the opportunity cost of capital. When reporting costs, they should always be reported in the same year, i.e. adjusting for the effects of inflation.

The cost of other related services includes the staffing, supplies, overheads and capital costs associated with community, ambulance and voluntary services. For example, the introduction of day-case surgery may seem

Table 3.3   Discount factors and equivalent annual costs of £1 per year for a discount rate of 6% (base year = year 0)

Year(s)	Discount factor (= present value of £1)	Equivalent annual cost of £1
1	0.9434	1.0600
2	0.8900	0.5454
3	0.8396	0.3741
4	0.7921	0.2886
5	0.7473	0.2374
6	0.7050	0.2034
7	0.6651	0.1791
8	0.6274	0.1610
9	0.5919	0.1470
10	0.5584	0.1359
11	0.5268	0.1268
12	0.4970	0.1193
13	0.4688	0.1130
14	0.4423	0.1076
15	0.4173	0.1030
16	0.3936	0.0989
17	0.3714	0.0954
18	0.3503	0.0924
19	0.3305	0.0896
20	0.3118	0.0872
21	0.2942	0.0850
22	0.2775	0.0830
23	0.2618	0.0813
24	0.2470	0.0797
25	0.2330	0.0782
26	0.2198	0.0769
27	0.2074	0.0757
28	0.1956	0.0746
29	0.1846	0.0736
30	0.1741	0.0726
31	0.1643	0.0718
32	0.1550	0.0710
33	0.1561	0.0703
34	0.1379	0.0696
35	0.1301	0.0690
36	0.1227	0.0684
37	0.1158	0.0679
38	0.1092	0.0674
39	0.1031	0.0670
40	0.0972	0.0665
41	0.0917	0.0661
42	0.0865	0.0657
43	0.0816	0.0653
44	0.0770	0.0650
45	0.0727	0.0647
46	0.0685	0.0644
47	0.0647	0.0641
48	0.0610	0.0639
49	0.0575	0.0637
50	0.0543	0.0634

efficient from the hospital resource perspective. However, if day-case surgery is followed by a visit from the community nurse on the evening of the patient's discharge from hospital it is important to include this cost within an evaluation of day-case surgery as this may offset the predicted savings gained. These related services are valued as described above for staffing, consumables, overheads and capital costs. Voluntary services are often excluded from costing studies, the argument for this being that such services are provided 'free of charge' and therefore incur no costs. However, despite not having a monetary cost, such services still have an associated opportunity cost if the time spent doing voluntary work had an alternative use, whether that alternative be paid work, unpaid work or leisure (see below to see how to value the opportunity cost of time).

Depending on the perspective of the study, costs to patients, their families and their friends may also require inclusion in an evaluation. These costs may be in terms of both time and money. For example, time and money costs may be incurred in travelling to and from appointments and people may forego income in attending their appointment. Childminding costs may be incurred when staying in hospital or visiting the GP. When a relative or friend is required to care for an ill patient there is an associated opportunity cost as they may do so at the expense of a paid job or some leisure activity. Money costs incurred should be valued at the actual amount. The opportunity cost of time depends on the alternative use of this resource. If this is paid employment then the value is proxied as the average wage rate; for unpaid labour the value is currently proxied at 54% of the average wage rate and for leisure time the value is taken as 43% of the average wage rate (Department of Transport 1989).

Indirect costs consist of time lost from work and costs external to health and welfare services. For example, when comparing drug therapy with surgical treatment for a condition, the calculation of indirect costs would be important if the drug therapy meant the patient could continue to work while the surgical treatment required absence from work. Currently indirect costs are rarely included in economic evaluations of health-care programmes because they are difficult to identify and are often negligible (Drummond et al 1987, Ratcliffe 1995, Donaldson & Shackley 1997).

It is clear from Box 3.1 that there are numerous types of costs to include in an economic evaluation. Collecting such information may be both time consuming and expensive. A shortcut method, known as reduced list costing, may be used to generate research economies. Knapp & Beecham (1993) showed that by identifying a reduced list of services which accounts for the greater part of the total cost of care in mental health and by concentrating on these key services, the majority of costs can be predicted. However, Whynes & Walker (1995) show that whilst use of a reduced list is likely to generate substantial research economies, it may do so at the expense of accuracy.

Box 3.2   Key points in costing

- Always use opportunity cost as a reflection of 'cost'.
- Use marginal costs, not average cost of per diem costs, where possible.
- Discount costs arising in the future.
- Perform sensitivity analysis on any assumptions made.
- Annuitise capital costs.
- Avoid double counting.

Care should be taken to avoid double counting when collecting costing data. For example, when comparing two surgical techniques and detailed information has been collected on the resources used in the operating theatre such as staff and consumables, it must be remembered that when the hourly cost of an operating theatre is added this normally includes token amounts for items such as consumables and staffing. Thus, it would be important to 'purge' the theatre cost of those elements of staff and consumables already included so as to avoid double counting.

Box 3.2 provides a summary of the key points to consider when conducting a costing exercise.

BENEFIT ASSESSMENT

What do we mean by benefits from health care?

To date, benefit assessment has focused almost exclusively on health outcomes. Definitions of health outcome have varied, ranging from very narrow definitions such as distress and disability to broader definitions which take account of multiple attributes of health. Concentration on health outcome only, however, fails to allow for the possibility of individuals deriving benefit from non-health and process attributes (Gerard et al 1992, Mooney & Lange 1993, Mooney 1994, Ryan & Farrar 1999, Ryan 1995, Ryan 1999, Ryan et al 2000, Donaldson et al 1995). Non-health outcomes are sources of benefit such as the provision of information, reassurance, autonomy and dignity in the provision of care. Process attributes include such aspects of care as waiting time, location of treatment, continuity of care, staff attitudes. For example, in the provision of screening programmes (e.g. prenatal screening programmes or screening for breast or cervical cancer) individuals may derive utility from the information and reassurance from obtaining a true-negative result (Gerard et al 1992, Mooney & Lange 1993, Donaldson et al 1995). In the provision of new reproductive technologies (NRTs), individuals may gain utility from knowing they have done everything possible to have a child, even if they leave the service childless, and factors such as waiting time, staff attitudes and continuity of care may also be important in the process of care (Ryan 1995). With regard to the process of treatment, local clinics with longer waiting times may be preferred to central clinics with shorter waiting times (Ryan & Farrar 1999, Ryan & McIntool 2000).

Measuring benefits from health care

Alongside the debate about *what constitutes* benefits in health-care has been a debate concerning *how to measure* such benefits. This latter question obviously depends on the answer to the former. That is, only when we know what it is we want to measure can we decide how to measure it.

Clinical measures of outcome

Initial attempts to measure benefits in health economics were very narrow. The outcome measure was clinical in nature and unidimensional, e.g. life years gained; pain reduction; cases detected; disability days avoided; and cholesterol reduction. Whilst relatively simple to measure, many important benefits may be ignored using this approach. For example, where life years are gained in a programme, the quality of such years may be important. Further, non-health outcomes and process attributes may also be important. These limitations have led to the development of other measures for benefit assessment.

Quality-adjusted life years (QALYs)

QALYs were developed to take account of the fact that people may be concerned with the quality of their lives as well as their length of life. To estimate QALYs, the expected number of life years gained from given health-care interventions are estimated (usually by health-care professionals) and combined with information on the quality of these life years (via the estimation of utility or quality weights). For example, if a health-care intervention results in a health state with a quality weight of 0.85 and the individual would be in this health state for the remainder of life, say 10 years, then the number of (undiscounted) QALYs would be 8.5. If the number of QALYs without the intervention were 4, then the QALYs gained from the intervention would be 4.5 (8.5 – 4). The QALYs gained from one health-care intervention may be compared with QALYs obtained from alternative health-care interventions, as well as from doing nothing. There are two main steps in the QALY framework: deciding what health outcome attributes to value and thereafter attaching utility weights to these outcomes.

Attributes in the QALY framework.   Generic measures of utility refer to utility indexes designed to measure attributes of health outcome that are held to be relevant to many types of illnesses and diseases. The original generic QALY proposed two dimensions of health outcome: distress and disability (Williams 1985). More recently the EuroQol has been developed (EuroQol 1990, Kind et al 1994, Williams 1995). This takes a more multidimensional approach than the Rosser Matrix, with five attributes: mobility; self-care; usual activities; pain/discomfort; and anxiety/depression.

The Short Form 36 (SF-36) is an increasingly widely used generic measure of health status in health service research (Ware & Sherbourne 1992). It consists of eight dimensions of health: physical functioning; physical role functioning; bodily pain; general health; vitality; social functioning; emotional role functioning; and mental health. Recently the instrument has been considered in the health economics literature as a potential generic health classification system and attempts are being made to define possible health outcomes in terms of a single utility score for use in economic evaluations (Brazier et al 1998).

Generic measures of health outcome have been criticised for being too narrow and insensitive to the outcomes of specific conditions. For example, Donaldson et al (1988) show that the use of generic QALYs in assessing the benefits of long-term care for elderly people is not sufficiently sensitive to changes in the relevant dimensions. They argue that more condition-specific measures are required. Examples of condition-specific measures include the Arthritis Impact Measuring Scale (AIMS) which was developed to assess the physical, emotional and social well-being of patients with rheumatic conditions; the Functional Living Index-Cancer (FLIC) and QL-Index which were developed specifically for use with cancer patients; and the Barthel Index as a single measure of independence in chronically ill patients. For more details on specific health status measures, see Walker & Rosser (1993).

Establishing utility weights. Once important attributes have been identified, utility weights need to be attached to the various possible outcomes. The three most common methods of establishing weights are: visual analogue; standard gamble; and time trade-off.

Visual Analogue Scale (VAS). Using this method, respondents are presented with possible outcomes of a health-care intervention and asked to place these along a physical line to reflect their relative ranking (Nord 1991). The relative distance between their placing is also meant to reflect respondents' relative preferences for the outcomes. Zero is usually taken to be the worst outcome (death) and 1 the best (full health). The utility weight is taken as the point at which the outcome is placed on the line. This method is not popular with economists since it does not incorporate any notion of sacrifice. As noted earlier, in economics, something only has value if a sacrifice is made for it.

Standard gamble (SG). This technique asks respondents to sacrifice 'certainty' in valuing a health outcome. Utility weights are estimated by presenting an individual with a number of paired comparisons in which they must choose between a certain outcome (B) or a gamble which may

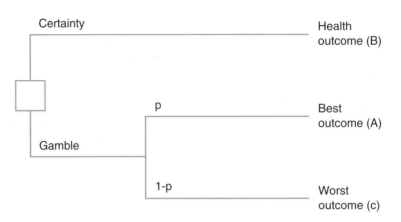

Certainty — Health outcome (B)

p — Best outcome (A)

Gamble

1-p — Worst outcome (c)

Fig. 3.1 An example of a standard gamble question.

result in either a better outcome (A) than the certain outcome (with a probability p) or a worse outcome (C) than the certain outcome (with a probability $1-p$). The certain outcome is always an intermediate outcome in the sense that the better outcome is always preferred to it and the worse outcome is less preferred to it. The probability of the best outcome is varied until the individual is indifferent between the certain intermediate outcome and the gamble. This probability is the utility for the certain outcome (McNeil et al 1981). This technique is then repeated for all intermediate outcomes. Figure 3.1 shows the SG format.

It is clear that if the certain outcome (B) is undesirable then the individual will be willing to take a treatment gamble even if the probability of the best outcome is very low (A). Thus, the utility weight for outcome (B) would also be very low. Hence, using the SG technique, the more undesirable an outcome, the lower the probability that the individual will accept the gamble and the lower the utility weight for the undesirable outcome. The SG method can be difficult and time consuming to administer.

Time trade-off (TTO). The TTO technique has been developed as an alternative, and easier, method than SG for estimating utility weights (Torrance et al 1972). It is favoured by economists over the VAS as it embodies a notion of sacrifice, namely 'time'. The approach involves presenting individuals with a paired comparison between living for a period t in a specified but less than perfect state (outcome B) versus having a healthier life (outcome A) for a shorter time period h (where h is always less than t). Time h is varied until the respondent is indifferent between the alternatives. The utility weight given to the less than perfect state is then h/t. Using the TTO technique, the more undesirable outcome B (the outcome being assessed) is, the more years of life an individual would be willing to give up to be in the best outcome (A) and the lower

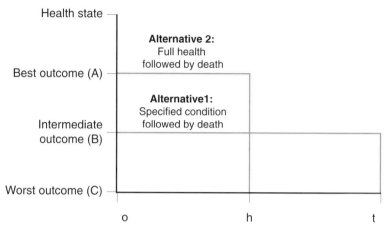

Fig. 3.2   An example of a time trade-off question.

the ratio h/t and in turn the utility of outcome B. Figure 3.2 shows the time trade-off technique.

Estimating QALYs.   The process of estimating QALYs is best explained with an example. Imagine that there are two possible treatments for sufferers of arthritis. One is the medical management of the disease and the other is a surgical intervention. Table 3.4 shows the two quality of life profiles for a 55-year-old woman for a period of 10 years. The profiles have been identified using the latest EuroQol descriptive system as presented in Box 3.3. The utility weights for these states of health have been calculated using the time trade-off technique and are presented in Table 3.5. Table 3.6 demonstrates the estimation of QALYs.

Whatever type of treatment the woman has, it is estimated that she will live a further 10 years. However, the type of treatment she receives will influence the quality of her life. If the woman has medical management,

Table 3.4   Quality of life outcomes from the EuroQol Descriptive System

Year	Quality of life level	
	Medical management	Surgical management
1	21111	22323
2	21111	12121
3	21111	12121
4	21111	12121
5	22121	12121
6	22121	12121
7	22121	12121
8	22121	12121
9	21323	22222
10	21323	22222

Box 3.3 The EuroQol Descriptive System (Dolan et al 1995)

Mobility
1. No problems in walking about
2. Some problems in walking about
3. Confined to bed

Self-care
1. No problems with self-care
2. Some problems washing or dressing self
3. Unable to wash or dress self

Usual activities
1. No problems with performing usual activities (e.g. work, study, housework, family or leisure activities)
2. Some problems with performing usual activities
3. Unable to perform usual activities

Pain/discomfort
1. No pain or discomfort
2. Moderate pain or discomfort
3. Extreme pain or discomfort

Anxiety/depression
1. Not anxious or depressed
2. Moderately anxious or depressed
3. Extremely anxious or depressed

Note: For convenience each composite health state has a five-digit code number relating to the relevant level of each dimension, with the dimension always listed in the order given above. Thus 11223 means:

   1 No problems in walking about
   1 No problems with self-care
   2 Some problems with performing usual activities
   2 Moderate pain or discomfort
   3 Extremely anxious or depressed

---

the first 5 years of her remaining 10 years will be spent in health state 21111 (with a quality weight of 0.87) and the last 5 years in health states 22121 and 21323 (with quality weights of 0.64 and 0.15). Discounting these quality weights (using the 6% rate), the total QALYs gained from medical management from no treatment is estimated to be 4.943. Surgical treatment gives rise to 4.511 discounted QALYs

Willingness to pay (WTP)

The technique of WTP is based on the premise that the maximum amount of money an individual is willing to pay (sacrifice) for a commodity is an indicator of the utility or satisfaction to them of that commodity. The most obvious market where WTP behaviour is revealed is auctions. Here individuals are pushed to consider the maximum amount of money they are willing to pay for a given commodity with given attributes. If the auction

Table 3.5 EuroQol utility scores

Health state	Utility score
21111	0.87
11211	0.87
11121	0.85
12111	0.83
11112	0.82
12211	0.76
12121	0.74
11122	0.72
22121	0.64
22112	0.66
11312	0.55
21222	0.55
12222	0.54
21312	0.51
22122	0.53
22222	0.50
11113	0.39
13212	0.38
13311	0.33
11131	0.20
12223	0.21
21323	0.15
23321	0.14
32211	0.14
21232	0.06
22323	0.04

Table 3.6 Using EuroQol to estimate the benefits from surgical and medical management for arthritis patients

Year	Discount factor*	Medical management		Surgical management	
		Utility	Discounted utility	Utility	Discounted utility
1	0.9434	0.87	0.821	0.04	0.038
2	0.8900	0.87	0.774	0.74	0.659
3	0.8396	0.87	0.730	0.74	0.621
4	0.7921	0.87	0.689	0.74	0.586
5	0.7473	0.64	0.478	0.74	0.553
6	0.7050	0.64	0.451	0.74	0.522
7	0.6651	0.64	0.426	0.74	0.492
8	0.6274	0.64	0.401	0.74	0.464
9	0.5919	0.15	0.089	0.5	0.296
10	0.5584	0.15	0.084	0.5	0.279
Total		6.34	**4.943**	6.22	**4.511**

* There is some controversy about whether to discount benefits at the same rate as costs. This example used a discount rate of 6%. For a summary of the discussion around this topic see Parsonage & Neuberger (1992) and Cairns (1992).

bid exceeds their maximum WTP, they will drop out. When deciding on maximum WTP, they will take account of the characteristics or attributes of the commodity that are important to them. For example, in a housing auction the individual will consider such characteristics as number of rooms, location, whether centrally heated, whether double glazed and house type. When an individual considers their maximum WTP they take account of all the attributes of the service of importance to them. Thus, using WTP to estimate the benefits of health-care should allow individuals to value health outcomes, non-health outcomes and process attributes.

WTP can be estimated using four techniques: open-ended; bidding; payment card; and closed-ended (for more information on these techniques, see Mitchell & Carson 1989). Using the open-ended technique, respondents are asked directly what is the maximum amount of money that they would be willing to pay for a commodity. If the WTP study is carried out via an interview, the bidding technique can be used. Here individuals are asked if they would be willing to pay a specified amount. If they answer 'yes', interviewers increase the bid until they reach amounts that the respondents are not willing to pay. If they answer 'no,' the interviewers lower the bid until they say 'yes'. WTP is estimated directly from the data provided. A variation on this is the payment card technique. Here respondents are presented with a range of bids and asked to circle the amount that represents the most they would be willing to pay. The individual's true maximum WTP will lie somewhere in the interval between the circled amount and the next highest option. The closed-ended (CE) approach asks individuals whether they would pay a specified amount for a given commodity, with possible responses being 'yes' or 'no'. The bid amount is varied across respondents and the only information obtained from each individual respondent is whether their maximum WTP is above or below the bid offered.

Estimating WTP. WTP was used by Ryan (1996a, 1997) to assess the value of assisted reproductive techniques (ARTs). Previous economic evaluations of ARTs were criticised for assuming that the only factor important to users is whether they leave the service with a child. That is, economic evaluations to date had estimated a cost per live birth, cost per maternity or cost per some other medical definition of success. Such an approach ignores, firstly, outcomes beyond some narrow medical definition of success (i.e. information, counselling and knowing you have done everything possible to have a child) and secondly, the majority of users who leave the service childless but who still experience outcomes beyond the clinical definition of success and thirdly, the actual process of treatment (i.e. waiting time, staff attitudes, continuity of care). The WTP approach would allow individuals to take account of all the above factors when valuing ARTs. Figure 3.3 shows examples of the open-ended, payment card and closed-ended WTP questions that were used in these studies. In one Australian study Ryan (1996a) used WTP to demonstrate that there was value in going through the service, even if the couple leave it childless. Taking account of all benefits, the value of ARTs to users was estimated to be AUS$2506 per attempt. In a study carried out in Aberdeen, Scotland, Ryan (1997) estimated that users had a mean value of over £5000 per attempt at ARTs.

Conjoint analysis (CA)

Conjoint analysis can be used to estimate utilities (for health outcomes, non-health outcomes and process attributes) and WTP. Whilst the technique is well established in the market research literature and widely used in

---

General information in all questions

In this section I am concerned with how you **value** IVF treatment

One way to do this is to find what the **maximum** amount of money is that you would be willing to pay for each IVF attempt you have. **You will not have to pay the amount you state. This is just a way of finding out how strongly you feel about IVF.**

Remember that any money you spend on IVF will not be available for you to spend on other things.

Example of open-ended WTP question

What is the **maximum** amount of money you would be willing to pay for your **current** attempt at IVF?

Remember that any money you spend on IVF will not be available for you to spend on other things

Maximum amount willing to pay for attempt £ _____

Example of open-ended question

Would you be willing to pay £ 2000* for your current attempt at IVF? (Please tick appropriate box.)

Yes ☐

No ☐

* Bid amount varied from £110 to £20,000

Fig. 3.3   Examples of WTP questions to value ARTs.

Example of payment card WTP question

Please consider whether you would be willing to pay each of the following amounts for your **current** IVF/GIFT attempt.

Remember that any money you spend on IVF/GIFT will not be available for you to spend on other things.

Willing to pay?

Amount per attempt	YES	NO
$0		
$300		
$550		
$750		
$1000		
$1300		
$1600		
$2000		
$2500		
$3000		
$3500		
$4000		
$4500		
$5000		
$7000		
$8000		
$10,000		

Please tick (√) YES if you are sure you would be willing to pay the amount

Please tick (√) NO if you are sure you would not be willing to pay the amount

*Please **circle** the maximum amount you would be willing to pay*

If you were willing to pay above $10,000 per attempt, please state the **maximum** amount of money you would be willing to pay $ _____

Fig. 3.3   Example of payment card WTP question. (Cont'd)

transport and environmental economics, it is only just beginning to be used in health economics (Propper 1995, Ryan 1995, 1996b, Ryan & Hughes 1997, Ryan 1999, Ryan et al 2000, Bryan et al 1998, Vick & Scott 1998, Van Der Pol & Cairns 1998). Its increased use in health economics can be partly explained by the need for a technique that can take account of more than health outcomes.

The initial stages of a CA study are similar to that of the QALY approach, i.e. establish what attributes are important and what levels to give to them. The technique differs from the QALY framework in the way preferences are elicited. Using CA, preferences may be elicited using ranking rating or discrete choice exercises. The approach currently favoured by economists is the discrete choice approach, partly because it incorporates the notion of sacrifice. Here the individual is asked to make numerous choices between two options, A and B, which may vary with regard to health attributes, non-health attributes and process attributes or any combination of these. Regression techniques are used to analyse the responses and both utilities and WTP can be estimated from the output.

Estimating utilities and WTP.   Conjoint analysis was used by Ryan (1999) to look at the value of alternative attributes of ARTs. The type of question respondents face is shown in Figure 3.4. The results from the regression analysis are shown in Table 3.7. The second column shows the coefficients from the regression output and the third column the marginal WTP for each of these attributes. Marginal WTP is estimated by dividing the relevant coefficient by the coefficient on cost. Utility and WTP for different types of IVF clinics can be estimated by looking at the differences from, say, the current system to a proposed alternative. In the example in Table 3.7, this would result in a utility score of 0.868 and a WTP of £1894. (For more information on the analysis and interpretation of CA see Ryan (1996b), Ryan & Hughes (1997) and Ryan et al (2000).)

Box 3.4 provides a summary of the key points to consider when conducting a benefit assessment exercise.

Choice 4	Clinic A	Clinic B
Attitudes of staff towards you	Good	Bad
Chance of taking home a baby	25%	35%
Continuity of contact with same staff	No	Yes
Time on waiting list for IVF attempt	18 months	18 months
Cost to you of IVF attempt	£1500	£3000
Follow-up support	No	No
Which clinic would you prefer *(tick one box only)*	Prefer Clinic A ☐	Prefer Clinic B ☐

Fig. 3.4   Example of discrete choice question in conjoint analysis questionnaire.

Box 3.4   Key points in benefit measurement

- Ideal economic measures of benefit incorporate some notion of sacrifice.
- Decide what it is you are trying to measure – only then can you decide what instrument to use.
- If potential benefits of a health-care intervention are not restricted to 'health gain' but include non-health outcomes and process attributes, a benefit measure which is sensitive to such factors should be used.
- Benefits occurring in the future should be discounted.
- Perform sensitivity analysis.

Table 3.7 Output from conjoint analysis study

Attribute	Coefficient	Marginal WTP (£)	Current	Proposed	Difference	Marginal utility	Marginal WTP
Process attributes							
Attitudes of staff towards you (0 = bad, 1 = good)	0.492*	1148	0	1	1	0.492	1148
Continuity of contact with same staff (0 = no, 1 = yes)	0.191*	445	0	1	1	0.191	445
Cost to you of IVF (£)	−0.0004*	n/a	1500	2000	500	−0.2	n/a
Time on waiting list for IVF (months)	−0.042*	97	6	3	−3	0.126	291
Health outcome							
Chance of taking home a baby (%)	0.077*	181	15	20	5	0.385	905
Non-health outcomes							
Follow-up support (0 = no, 1 = yes)	−0.187*	435	0	0	0	0	0
Total						0.868	1894

*Significant at 1% level

TECHNIQUES OF ECONOMIC EVALUATION

This section examines how the costs and benefits discussed in the previous sections can be brought together within the framework of an economic evaluation. The three principal economic evaluation techniques are: cost-benefit analysis (CBA), cost-effectiveness analysis (CEA) and cost-utility analysis (CUA). The technique(s) chosen will be determined by whether the question being addressed is concerned with allocative efficiency or technical efficiency. An allocative efficiency question is concerned with 'whether' to allocate resources to a given programme. All health-care programmes have to compete for scarce health-care resources. These 'competing' health-care programmes may include, for example, gynaecological services, intensive care services, oncology services, renal services and rheumatology. An allocative efficiency question would be: should there be an expansion of surgery for hernia repair or increased provision of rheumatology clinics? In contrast, technical efficiency is concerned with 'within programme' efficiency, i.e. how best to provide a given service. The resources, or budget allocated to a programme, are taken as given and the issue is simply 'how best' to provide that service. A technical efficiency question would be: when providing hernia repair surgery, is it best to provide conventional surgery or laparoscopic surgery? Or, when providing rheumatology clinics, is it best to provide a nurse practitioner service or a consultant-based service?

Cost-effectiveness analysis

Cost-effectiveness analysis (CEA) can only be used to address questions of technical efficiency. It examines the effects of at least two competing alternatives 'within a fixed budget'. A ratio for each alternative is provided, the numerator being cost and the denominator the health effect. Such effects are measured in unidimensional terms, i.e. life years saved, heart attacks prevented, percentage reduction in cholesterol concentration or improvement in limb function. The cost-effectiveness ratio produced is, therefore, a measure of 'cost per unit of effect'. The alternative with the lowest cost-effectiveness ratio, is the preferred choice.

The main limitation of CEA is that the unit of health effect must be unidimensional. Thus, only interventions with the same goal can be compared. Further, important effects may be excluded from analyses. For example, in some cancer therapies, while years of remaining life are an important outcome measure, the quality of those remaining years may be equally important. Similarly, non-health outcomes and process attributes may also be important.

The phrase 'within a given budget' is of crucial importance. Often authors produce a ratio of *extra* costs per *extra* unit of health effect of one intervention over another, calling this an incremental cost-effectiveness ratio (ICER). Such ratios are not CEAs. CEA, by definition, assumes that health effects should be maximised 'within a given budget' and that alternatives with the lowest cost-effectiveness ratio should be chosen. An ICER assumes that there are additional benefits for additional costs and this suggests that, since they are 'additional', these costs will come from outwith the fixed budget. Hence, given limited resources, some judgement is required as to whether such extra costs are worth incurring as they will have to be taken from some other programme. This takes us back to the broader issues of allocative efficiency, i.e. 'whether' to allocate, not 'how' to allocate. CEA cannot address such a question.

Cost-utility analysis

In health economics, cost-utility analysis (CUA) has become synonymous with the QALY framework. CUA can be seen as an improvement on CEA as it attempts to combine more than one outcome measure and takes account of both quality and quantity of life. One reason for the development of the QALY framework was to enable comparisons to be made across health-care interventions, i.e. so that allocative efficiency questions could be addressed. Such comparisons can only be made when generic QALYs are used, such that alternative health-care interventions can be compared on the same dimensions. Using QALYs for questions of allocative efficiency, marginal cost per additional QALY league tables are constructed. The number of QALYs achieved from a health-care budget will be maximised by allocating resources to those interventions with the lowest cost per QALY ratio.

CUA and cost per QALY ratios may also be used to address technical efficiency questions. Here programme-specific dimensions of quality of life may be used, as well as generic measures (the former cannot be used for questions of allocative efficiency). An example of the use of cost per QALY information within the context of a technical efficiency question is provided in Table 3.5. Here the question is whether to provide surgical or medical management for arthritis. Assuming a discounted cost of medical management of £3682 and a discounted cost of surgical management of £2830 and using the discounted benefits estimated above, the cost per QALY is £745 for medical management and £627 for surgical management. Given that the number of QALYs achieved from a fixed budget will be maximised by allocating resources to those interventions with the lowest cost per QALY ratio, the optimal treatment is surgical management.

QALY league tables have been criticised on a number of grounds (Gerard & Mooney 1993). Three main problems have been identified: the relevant measure of cost in QALY league tables has to be restricted to health service resource use; the relevant measure of benefit in QALY league tables is clearly restricted to health outcomes; and the legitimacy of transferring marginal costs and benefits to different settings is debatable. Donaldson & Shackley (1997) also note that there is a question of whether the original context of the study will allow the results to be transferred to the local context of the decision maker as each item in the league table has a different comparator. The cost per QALY gained in programme A may have been produced by comparing programme A with programme B. However, if B is inefficient to begin with, A may be inefficient too. Yet, even if A is inefficient, it may still look good because it was compared with B (another inefficient programme).

Whilst CUA has become synonymous with QALYs, the technique can be broadened to include measures of utility that take account of health outcomes, non-health outcomes and process attributes. Rather than estimate a cost per QALY, a cost per 'util' would be estimated. Utilities could be estimated using conjoint analysis (as demonstrated above). This approach is in its infancy in health economics and further research is needed to look at how utility scores estimated from conjoint analysis studies can be used to address technical efficiency and allocative efficiency questions.

Cost-benefit analysis

Cost-benefit analysis (CBA) is commonly used to address allocative efficiency, though it can also be used to address technical efficiency. It requires all costs and benefits to be measured in commensurate units, usually money. Costs can then be directly compared with benefits. CBA is the only form of evaluation which directly addresses the question of whether a particular intervention is 'worthwhile', i.e. whether the benefits of a programme or intervention exceed its cost. Benefits are traditionally measured using either the human capital approach or the WTP approach. The human capital approach values health improvements on the basis of future productive worth to society resulting from being able to return to work (paid or unpaid). There are a number of problems with this approach and it is now widely accepted that the alternative WTP approach is theoretically superior and hence preferred (Drummond et al 1987).

Very few CBA studies have been carried out in the field of health-care, despite the titles of many articles bearing the name (Donaldson & Shackley 1997). Many cost-benefit studies often turn out to be a comparison of costs incurred and savings accrued. However, this clearly involves only a comparison of costs with no consideration of the valuation of health benefits in monetary terms (Donaldson & Shackley 1997). Despite the problems with CBA, it remains a useful framework for setting out a decision-making problem. By identifying the costs and benefits associated with alternative health-care interventions or programmes and valuing what can be valued, the trade-offs between costs and benefits are made explicit.

One example of a CBA is a study by Ryan (1997) which addressed the issue of whether government should fund assisted reproductive techniques (ARTs). Benefits of ARTs were assessed using the closed-ended WTP technique to establish the value the infertile place on in vitro fertilisation (IVF) treatment in Scotland. The results suggested an average WTP of users for ARTs of £5000 per attempt. This compared with a cost of £2700.

When using the results of WTP studies in CBA, it is important to note that the decision rule will depend on the context in which the questions are asked. The conventional use of WTP values is to provide a service when WTP is greater than costs, i.e. where the benefit/cost ratio is greater than 1. When a good is privately provided this rule is acceptable. Thus, in relation to the above example, if provision of ARTs is being considered in the private sector, then the results suggest that the benefits of the service outweigh the costs and that the provision of the service should be encouraged. However, this decision rule may not be appropriate in the public sector, such as the NHS, where there is a fixed budget and where many competing health-care interventions may have a benefit/cost ratio greater than 1. The problem here is that more health-care interventions may have a benefit/cost ratio greater than 1 than can be provided by the limited budget. Thus, whilst the benefits of ARTs are greater than their costs, this may also be the case for many other health-care interventions. For a more detailed discussion of this see Shackley & Donaldson (1997).

CONCLUSION

By outlining the concepts of scarcity, choice and opportunity cost and their relevance to health-care, this chapter has provided an introduction to the issues surrounding economic evaluation in health care. The methods for measuring and valuing costs and benefits have been outlined and the methods by which the costs and benefits are collated within an economic evaluation technique have been described. This chapter has placed particular emphasis on the techniques for measuring and valuing the benefits in health-care evaluation as this can be seen as the most challenging area in health-care evaluation. By incorporating relatively new techniques in health-care evaluation such as WTP and CA and drawing on examples from the literature, this chapter aims to highlight the areas where future research will concentrate. Research has shown that patients place 'value' on other non-health and process attributes such as reassurance, information, attitudes of staff and waiting time and techniques such as WTP and CA allow consideration of these factors.

Economic evaluation should be seen as a decision-making framework which renders explicit the costs and benefits of any intervention or service. In doing so, informed decisions can be made about the allocation of resources to various programmes. The outcome or benefit measure chosen will decide the actual 'type' of economic evaluation carried out. If a number of outcome measures are chosen, a variety of economic evaluations may be performed and the results used as an aid to decision making. Ensuring that the opportunity costs of programmes are minimised should ensure the maximisation of well-being in society given limited resources.

Acknowledgements

The Health Economics Research Unit is funded by the Chief Scientist Office of the Scottish Office Department of Health (SODoH). The views expressed in this chapter are those of the authors, not SODoH. The authors are grateful to Phil Shackley for comments on earlier drafts of this chapter.

REFERENCES

Brazier J, Usherwood T, Harper R, Thomas K 1998 Deriving a preference-based single index from the UK SF-36 Health Survey. Journal of Clinical Epidemiology 51: 1115–1128

Briggs A, Sculpher M, Buxton M 1994 Uncertainty in the economic evaluation of health care technologies: the role of sensitivity analysis. Health Economics 3: 95–104

Bryan S, Baxter M, Sheldon R, Grant A 1998 Magnetic resonance imaging for the investigation of knee injuries: an investigation of preferences. Health Economics 7: 595–603

Cairns J 1992 Discounting and health benefits: another perspective. Health Economics 1: 76–79

Department of Transport 1989 Values of time and vehicle operating costs for 1989. COBA 9 Manual, Annex II, section 8.2.8.3–8.10. Department of Transport, London

Dolan P, Gudex C, Kind P, Williams A 1995 A social tariff for EuroQol: results from a UK general population survey. Discussion paper no. 138, Centre for Health Economics, University of York, York

Donaldson C, Shackley P 1997 Economic evaluation. In: Detels R, Holland W, McEwan J, Omenn G (eds) Oxford textbook of public health, 3rd edn. Oxford University Press, Oxford, pp. 849–871

Donaldson C, Atkinson A, Bond J 1988 Should QALYs be programme specific? Journal of Health Economics 7: 239–257

Donaldson C, Shackley P, Abdalla M, Miedzybrodzka Z 1995 Willingness to pay for antenatal carrier screening for cystic fibrosis. Health Economics 4: 439–452

Drummond M F, Stoddart G L, Torrance W 1987 Methods for the economic evaluation of health care programmes. Oxford University Press, Oxford

EuroQol 1990 EuroQol – a new facility for the measurement of health-related quality of life. Health Policy 16: 199–208

Gerard K, Mooney G 1993 QALY league tables: handle with care. Health Economics 2: 59–64

Gerard K, Turnbull D, Lange M, Mooney G 1992 Economic evaluation of mammography screening: information, reassurance and anxiety. Health Economics Research Unit discussion paper no. 01/92. University of Aberdeen, Aberdeen

Jacobs P, Baladi J F 1996 Biases in cost measurement for economic evaluation studies in health care. Health Economics 5: 525–529

Kind P, Dolan P, Gudex C, Williams A 1994 Practical and methodological issues in the development of the EuroQol: the York experience. Advances in Medical Sociology 5: 219–253

Knapp M, Beecham J 1993 Reduced list costings: examination of an informed short cut in mental health research. Health Economics 2: 313–322

McNeil B, Weichselbaum R, Stephen G, Pauker G 1981 Speech and survival. New England Journal of Medicine 305: 982–987

Mitchell R C, Carson R T 1989 Using surveys to value public goods. Resources for the Future, Washington DC

Mooney G 1994 What else do we want from our health services? Social Science and Medicine 39: 151–154

Mooney G, Lange M 1993 Ante-natal screening: what constitutes benefit? Social Science and Medicine 37: 873–878

Neuhauser D, Lewicki A M 1975 What do we gain from the sixth stool guaiac? New England Journal of Medicine 293: 255–258

Nord E 1991 The validity of a visual analogue scale in determining social utility weight for health states. International Journal of Health Planning and Management 6: 234–242

Parsonage M, Neuberger H 1992 Discounting and health benefits. Health Economics 1: 71–79

Propper C 1995 The disutility of time spent on the United Kingdom's National Health Service waiting lists. Journal of Human Resources 30: 677–700

Ratcliffe J 1995 The measurement of indirect costs in economic evaluation: a critical review. Project Appraisal 10: 13–18

Ratcliffe J, Ryan M, Tucker J 1996 The costs of alternative types of routine antenatal care for low risk women: shared care vs care by general practitioners and community midwives. Journal of Health Services Research and Policy 1: 135–140

Ryan M 1995 Economics and the patient's utility function: an application to Assisted Reproductive Techniques. PhD thesis, University of Aberdeen, Aberdeen

Ryan M 1996a Using willingness to pay to assess the benefits of assisted reproductive techniques. Health Economics 5: 543–558

Ryan M 1996b Using consumer preferences in health care decision making: the application of conjoint analysis. Office of Health Economics, London

Ryan M 1997 Should government fund assisted reproductive techniques? A pilot study using willingness to pay. Applied Economics 29: 841–849

Ryan M 1999 A role for conjoint analysis in technology assessment in health care? International Journal of Technology Assessment in Health Care 15: 433–457

Ryan M, Farrer S 2000 Using conjoint analysis to elicit preferences for health care. British Medical Journal (in press)

Ryan M, Hughes J 1997 Using conjoint analysis to assess women's preferences for miscarriage management. Health Economics 6: 261–273

Ryan M, McIntosh E, Dean T, Old P 2000 Trade off between location and waiting times in the provision of health care: the case of elective surgery on the Isle of Wight. Journal of Public Health Medicine (in press)

Ryan M, Ratcliffe J, Tucker J 1997 Using willingness to pay to value alternative models of antenatal care. Social Science and Medicine 44: 371–380

Shackley P, Donaldson C 1997 Willingness to pay for collectively financed care. University of Sheffield, Sheffield

Torrance G, Thomas W, Sackett D 1972 A utility maximization model for evaluation of health care programs. Health Services Research 7: 118–133

Van Der Pol M, Cairns J 1998 Establishing patient preferences for blood transfusion support: an application of conjoint analysis. Journal of Health Services Research and Policy 3(2): 70–76

Vick S, Scott A 1998 What makes a perfect agent? A pilot study of patients' preferences in the doctor–patient relationship. Journal of Health Economics 17: 587–606

Ware J, Sherbourne C 1992 The SF-36 short-form health status survey 1. Conceptual framework and item selection. Medical Care 30: 473–483

Walker S, Rosser R 1993 Quality of life assessment: key issues in the 1990s. Kluwer Academic Publishers, Dordrecht

Whynes D K, Walker A R 1995 On approximations in treatment costing. Health Economics 4: 31–39

Williams A 1985 Economics of coronary artery bypass grafting. British Medical Journal 291: 326–329

Williams A 1995 The role of the EuroQol instrument in QALY calculations. Centre for Health Economics, York

FURTHER READING

Donaldson C, Shackley P 1997 Economic evaluation. In: Detels R, Holland W, McEwan J, Omenn G (eds) Oxford textbook of public health, 3rd edn. Oxford University Press, Oxford, pp. 849–871

Drummond M F, Stoddart G L, Torrance W 1987 Methods for the economic evaluation of health care programmes. Oxford University Press, Oxford

Mitchell R C, Carson R T 1989 Using surveys to value public goods. Resources for the Future, Washington DC

Ryan M 1996 Using consumer preferences in health care decision making: the application of conjoint analysis. Office of Health Economics, London

4

Information systems for public health nursing

John Womersley

INTRODUCTION

Unlike the hospital situation, there is no standard recording/information system for the community. The primary objective of an information system for public health nursing should be to provide information about health and social care needs for individuals and for population subgroups; it should not be used for monitoring activity or for justifying the role of the nurses. Nurses working in the community are in a unique position to form a very useful assessment of need. For example, by aggregating data for individuals, it is possible to assess need for a wide variety of population subgroups on a general practice, postcode area, client group or diagnostic basis.

This chapter sets out the potential contribution of community nurses to public health information systems. It details a proposed method of recording the information that community nurses often have at their fingertips, which at present is passed on only by word of mouth, in the absence of a relevant system.

To put nursing information in context with other NHS information systems, the chapter begins with a brief history of the use of statistics by health services and compares hospital and community information systems.

THE EVOLUTION OF HEALTH INFORMATION SYSTEMS

Lively debate about the health of populations and variations between and within populations flourished between about 1830 and the end of the 19th century. During that period new methods of recording and analysis were established, new techniques of presentation such as mapping came into use and the associations between ill health and a wide variety of demographic, socioeconomic and environmental factors were investigated in detail (Womersley 1987). Information was not collected for its own sake but as a crucial instrument for effecting social reform. The 19th-century health statisticians argued fiercely for improved standards of ventilation, housing, nutrition, clothing and cleanliness. For example, Robert Cowan (1840) proposed the establishment of a 'medical police' to help resolve problems such as 'recklessness and the use of ardent spirits' and suggested improvements in local government and in the provision of hospital services. Robert Perry (1844) used maps and vivid but horrifying reports from his district surgeons to demonstrate the need for boards of health in every town and city to help prevent the onset and spread of infectious disease and advocated setting a tax for the improvement of poor relief.

The methods used by these early analysts were often as sophisticated as any we have today. Thus the first medical officers of health (MOHs) in Glasgow and Edinburgh were able to collate information from a variety of sources for geographical areas as small as census enumeration districts of about 150 households or even for individual streets. It was Gairdner's (unfulfilled) ambition for the registrar to tabulate his returns for each enumeration district weekly, in order to 'afford instant information of the rise of the death rate, and to enable precautions to be specially directed to that quarter' (Womersley 1987). He envisaged that such returns would also be useful for identifying the causes 'of that permanent excess of mortality which we know to exist' and to discover to what extent this was dependent 'on faults in the arrangement of families, the construction of houses, overcrowding, deficient comforts, poverty, and so forth'.

Compelling statistics combined with forceful advocacy provided the impetus for the considerable improvements in housing and sanitation which took place towards the end of the 19th century. Almost at the end of the century, community nursing services began to be established in major cities, with the principal objectives of reducing infant mortality and improving maternal and child health and well-being in those areas where need was greatest. Shortly afterwards, concern about the health of army recruits during the Boer War led to a number of reports which promoted the idea that the state should be concerned not only with the removal of specific conditions inimical to health but should also accept responsibility for measures to promote health. These reports recommended routine medical inspection in schools and emphasised the opportunity provided by schools for taking stock of the physique of the whole population and securing the conditions most favourable to healthy development. Also during this period, systems were introduced for the notification of infectious disease (1889) and for notification of births by midwives (1907), this latter probably being the first public health measure taken not exclusively for protecting the community against spread of disease or for humanitarian reasons but for protecting the next and future generations.

By this time, annual reports on the health of their populations were being produced by MOHs for cities and major towns. In the early years these reports often reached a high standard of excellence, with detailed analyses of all-cause and cause-specific mortality rates together with demographic and socioeconomic indicators, particularly relating to housing, for small areas, usually municipal wards. In later years this detail was often omitted and the reports are generally less useful as sources of data and have poorer analytical commentary. The reports ceased with the demise of MOHs after 1974 and it was not until the late 1980s that health authorities again began to publish regular annual reports on the health of their populations and subgroups within them.

The lengthy break, from 1974 until almost 1990, in the reports on the health of populations coincided curiously with a period of remarkable growth in the development of information systems about hospital activity and with a massive increase in data processing and analytical power. Unfortunately, the huge resources committed to these developments were directed almost entirely to developing increasingly sophisticated computer systems with much less thought being given to how the information could be used to greater benefit or even to whether the data were at all accurate in the first place. The whole edifice was based on a most insecure foundation of relatively underpaid and otherwise demotivated records staff who had little understanding of what they were recording or why. Towards the end of this period, general practice microcomputer-based information systems also reached a stage of development where information about morbidity and risk factors could be recorded and readily analysed; however, except for a fairly limited data set required for population screening/surveillance purposes, extensive use of this capability was made only by a relatively small number of general practitioner enthusiasts.

Major changes in the organisation of the health service during the early 1990s, particularly fundholding, the new general practitioner contract and creation of the 'internal market', together with ever-increasing concern about costs have, in the hospital service, led to considerable improvements in the completeness and accuracy of much of the recorded data and to much greater and more imaginative use. General practice systems have also continued to develop. It is intended that all practices in the UK will form a network capable of linking to other sectors within the health service. This network is currently well advanced but there is quite a lot of technical work still to do before the more interesting issue of actually using it is addressed. Initially, only a minority of practices will fully exploit the public health uses of their computers and information systems but in time, the majority will probably reach the level of sophistication currently achieved by only the most forward looking. The one area in which virtually no progress appears to be being made in the development of effective information systems is that of community health services.

HOSPITAL AND COMMUNITY INFORMATION SYSTEMS COMPARED

Both hospital and general practice information systems generally focus on individual patients, although hospital systems relate to episodes of care which can be linked for each patient only with some difficulty. The nightly 'bed counts' which still take place in hospitals provide numeric data on occupancy levels, lengths of stay and throughput but for most analyses, more detailed information for each individual discharged is required.

Unlike the hospital and general practice systems, community information systems, and community nursing systems in particular, have focused on the activities of professional staff rather than on the characteristics and problems of the patients or on the value of any interventions. The emphasis in the community has been on developing computer systems and an obsessional desire to record every intervention at every patient contact rather than focusing on the problems and needs of patients and the extent to which these are being successfully managed.

Information systems have failed not only community nursing but also public health in general. Three important factors have contributed to this. First, community nurses themselves often wish to record every intervention they make, apparently as a means of justifying their role; this has led to unreasonable amounts of time being spent on recording data. Second, managers appear to want the same detail so that they can count contacts, procedures and visits and thereby produce copious but generally meaningless 'statistics' as a basis for formulating and 'monitoring' contracts. And third, those who design information systems often appear more concerned with technology, for example computer systems or particular methods of data entry such as optical mark/character recognition, than with defining what a meaningful community/public health information system should comprise. As a result, in contrast to the situation with hospitals, information systems for community health services have generally not evolved far beyond the stage of simplistic numeric computation.

The failure of community nurses and other health service professionals who work in the community to move beyond the collection and analysis of numbers to provide information on a population basis is a major missed opportunity. Community nurses, and particularly health visitors, are in a uniquely strong position to assess the health and identify the health and social care needs of defined populations and to monitor the progress or otherwise of patients after discharge from hospital.

In addition, it has not been generally realised that information about individuals in the community can readily be aggregated, on a geographic, client group, diagnostic or general practice basis, to form assessments of the health and needs of defined populations and of subgroups such as those living in particular localities, elderly people, ethnic minorities, people with physical disability, the terminally ill or those with a particular diagnostic condition. Such assessments would be invaluable to health boards/authorities and social service departments and would do a great deal more to enhance the role and reputation of community nurses than recording the details of every intervention.

THE DIVERSE RESPONSIBILITIES OF COMMUNITY NURSES

The responsibilities of community nurses range from technical tasks (mainly the responsibility of district nurses), which can be measured fairly readily, to less well-defined tasks such as prevention or promoting lifestyle change which are influenced by many factors apart from nursing interventions (see Box 4.1 for examples). The process of evaluating this more complicated activity is difficult and only likely to be achieved over a long period of time. It is also often difficult to attribute a successful outcome solely to intervention by individual community nurses.

This wide range of responsibilities places community nursing at the centre of a complex network of public health services (Fig. 4.1) comprising a variety of people in both statutory and voluntary agencies. Its general practice base provides responsibility for a defined population and its links with social services, voluntary organisations and (through liaison workers) hospitals enable the profession to facilitate the coordination of a wide range of support services. Box 4.2 illustrates the kind of information which, by virtue of their responsibilities and contacts, community nurses could potentially provide about the people and populations they serve.

WHAT CAN COMMUNITY NURSES CONTRIBUTE TO ASSESSMENT OF THE NEEDS OF THE POPULATION?

We have shown that by virtue of their contact with patients, their carers and families, the general practitioner, a wide variety of health and social service professionals and voluntary organisations, community nurses are in a unique position to assess the health and understand the health and social care needs of individuals. By aggregating data recorded about each individual (e.g. dates of birth, postcode, client group, diagnosis, physical/mental/social functioning), together with significant information about interventions and their outcome for those who have ongoing requirements for health care, it is possible to form a very useful assessment of needs for a wide variety of

Box 4.1 Some responsibilities of community nurses

Health surveillance (e.g. of preschool children, people with disabilities and special needs and people aged 75 years and over)
Identification of:
- those with health problems, social problems and other special needs
- those who have not had adequate health surveillance
- those who have not received appropriate treatment/interventions
- those who have not received necessary services.

Screening
Identification of:
- those who have not had a cervical and breast screening examination
- patients with risk factors for IHD, stroke and cancers.

Patient education and support
Evaluation of programmes such as:
- chronic disease management, e.g. for asthma, epilepsy, diabetes
- population health promotion, e.g. for healthy lifestyles, increasing social integration and self-esteem
- encouraging physically disabled and elderly patients to attain as near as possible their maximum potential in physical, mental and social functioning
- helping patients regain as much physical functioning as possible following events such as stroke, fracture and myocardial infarction
- follow-up and support after discharge from hospital in order to maximise potential for recovery and minimise need for readmission
- ensuring maximum possible control for people on medication for conditions such as diabetes, asthma, Parkinson's disease and epilepsy
- teaching what symptoms patients should react to and those which are self-limiting
- encouragement of self-examination for cancer of breasts, skin and testes
- supporting families through stress, including coping with new babies, bereavement, etc.

Immunisation
- Identification of children who are not fully immunised.

Elderly people and people with long-term physical disability
- Ensuring that physically disabled people of all ages whose disability is reduced by maximising mental or physical function or by external means (aids, appliances and functional support) are identified and offered appropriate assistance.
- Providing help and support for carers and families.

Advocacy
- *For individuals*, e.g. by provision of information, securing support (including financial help), involving patients and carers in decisions relating to health-care provision.
- *For groups*, e.g. by community development, informing purchasers, informing local and national government, promoting home care as a viable alternative to institutional care.
- *For public health*, e.g. traffic, water fluoridation.

subgroups within the population. Information can be made available on a variety of bases: by general practice; by postcode area (geographic area, ward or locality); by client group; and by diagnostic group. For self-limiting conditions only a minimum amount of data is necessary; for example, in order to identify variations in the need for, or provision of, community services after discharge from acute hospital. However, for people with

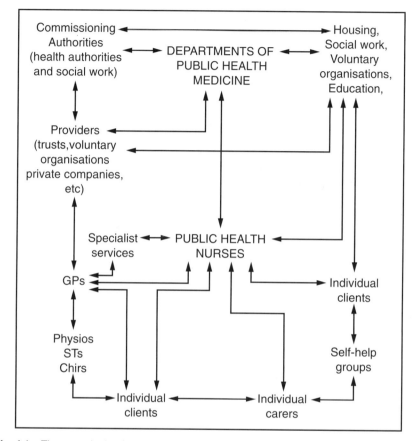

Fig. 4.1   The central role of the public health nurse in assessing the need for and coordinating health care.

long-term conditions or in particular client groups it is important to know not only their numbers but also, for example, their health-care and other needs, the extent to which these needs are being met, the quantity of input from health services, the objectives of such interventions, the extent to which these objectives are achieved and (for some groups) functional status and quality of life.

The number of population subgroups for which it is possible to aggregate data for individuals is almost limitless and includes those in a specific demographic group (e.g. preschool children, elderly people, ethnic minorities) or socioeconomic group, those living in a particular locality or those with a particular diagnostic condition or other characteristic (e.g. physical or mental disability). Clearly, it is possible to focus on only a small number of such subgroups at any one time and different issues will vary in importance at different times. It is important to be able to extend the ranges of information

---

Box 4.2 The type of information needed from community nursing information systems

For a general practice, ward, postcode sector, locality or client/diagnostic group

- How many wheelchair users, stroke patients, multiple sclerosis, Parkinson's, spina bifida and cystic fibrosis sufferers? What are their needs? Where do they live?
- What is the quality of life of residents of residential and nursing homes?
- What are the requirements for special needs housing?
- Are all those eligible receiving attendance allowance and other benefits?
- What is the effectiveness of our rehabilitation services?
- How satisfactory are responses to screening procedures (e.g. for cervical and breast cancer, hearing and visual deficiency and postnatal depression); to surveillance of preschool children, elderly people, asthmatics and diabetics; and to immunisation and other preventive services?
- Has there been any increase in breast feeding, reduction in childhood accidents or increase in smoking cessation in pregnant/postpartum mothers?
- Has there been an improvement in uptake of services and financial benefits by elderly people and those with long-term disabilities?
- Is there satisfactory early detection and appropriate management of potentially remediable health and social problems in children and elderly people?
- Is achievement in physically disabled and elderly people (including those living in nursing and residential homes) as near as possible to maximum potential in physical, mental and social functioning?
- Is there ready access to specialist help in the community for people suffering from long-term disabilities such as continence problems, multiple sclerosis, Parkinson's disease, epilepsy and dementia?
- Has there been any reduction in admission rates to hospital and long-term institutional care for conditions which could be successfully managed at home?
- Is it possible to reduce length of stay in hospital by ensuring that effective arrangements for community care are in place as soon as the patient is medically fit for discharge or to similarly achieve a reduction in the rates of readmission to hospital?
- Is it possible to demonstrate any improvement in quality of life for people suffering from long-term disorders and their carers and for those living in nursing and residential homes?

---

recorded about individuals in specific target groups for a limited time period for more in-depth analysis. For example, community nurses may wish to identify the unmet health and social care needs of people with learning difficulties; people living in a particularly deprived area or single-parent families; or they may wish to investigate ways of improving the care of people with epilepsy or of homeless families; or a specific problem such as a low breast-feeding rate, depression in older people or high smoking prevalence may be identified. Community nurses, with their extensive knowledge of community networks, are in an ideal position to involve members of the group in question in the process of need identification. Following need identification, community nurses then become involved in organising health promotion and other interventions and in evaluating the outcome.

Health and social care are at present organised as separate services in the UK, although they are organised in one agency in Northern Ireland. It could be argued that this is an unreasonable split and there is evidence to suggest that integration of the two services is both more effective and more efficient (Down Lisburn Trust 1994). Movement towards sharing information about individual clients between the two authorities is beginning to take place and politicians have recently indicated that some form of integration is under active consideration. It would seem reasonable, therefore, that any developments in information systems for community nurses should embrace social as well as health-care and that the totality of 'care' should be addressed by both social work and health professionals rather than its separate components.

TIME FOR COMMUNITY NURSES TO TAKE THE LEAD IN DEVELOPING THEIR INFORMATION SYSTEMS?

Community nurses in general spend a great deal of time recording data, much of which is processed by computer. Often, very little benefit is derived from this expensive activity because there is insufficient clarity about the reasons for collecting the data, with the emphasis being on data collection rather than on meaningful analysis. In addition, because little or no information is fed back to the nurses themselves, they become demotivated and the quality and accuracy of recording decline. Therefore, a complete culture change is needed, whereby community nurses themselves become the driving force for the development of information systems to assist them to carry out their responsibilities to maximum effect. The following principles may help the process of achieving this objective.

- The primary objective of any information system for community nurses should be to provide information about health and social care needs for individuals and population subgroups, not for monitoring the activities of the nurses.
- The nurses should receive regular analyses of the data which they record, with minimum delay; information should be provided for the nurses' own caseload, for relevant population subgroups and it should be possible to compare the characteristics of patients, for example between practitioners and between localities.
- Nurses should be able to obtain ad hoc analyses of public health nursing data on request and with minimal delay.
- Data that are not used should not be collected.
- The amount of data recorded for particular individuals should relate to the complexity of their needs and to the likely duration of their need for intervention. For people with only a short-term need for a relatively minor intervention, it is unnecessary to record any information on a

named-person basis. However, for people with complex care needs which are likely to persist, e.g. people with multiple sclerosis or learning difficulties, a detailed person-based record is needed so that the extent to which their needs are being met can be regularly monitored.

- Detailed information about process measures such as sources of referral, nature of interventions, referrals made, care hours, time between referral and intervention, outcome of referrals should be obtained only on a sample basis, say over one or two 1-week periods each year. This would reduce the recording of such details by 80–90% and would almost certainly increase interest and therefore improve levels of accuracy.
- Local groups of community nurses should be encouraged to use the information collected about individuals (e.g. ethnicity, single parenthood, smoking, breast feeding) as sampling frames for the conduct of more detailed investigations (e.g. of health/social care needs) and for the evaluation of interventions.

THREE LEVELS OF DATA RECORDING

The concept of recording the same detail for all contacts with patients/ clients on a continuing basis has far outlived its usefulness. A far more imaginative approach is required which includes special survey work and sampling procedures and which recognises that more detailed information is required about people with complex needs, with minimal or no detail for those whose needs are simple and short term. A three-tier system of data recording is suggested.

Level 1: basic recording

The great majority of patients have self-limiting conditions or require technical nursing such as an injection or dressing over a prolonged time period. Information about every patient contact or intervention is not necessary and should not be requested by managers. If required, these processes may be satisfactorily monitored on a sample basis, say over a 1- or 2-week period each year. There would be no need to identify individual patients; all that would be required is to record factors such as age, postcode, diagnosis, client group and nature of intervention.

Level 2: intermediate recording

For certain client groups it is important to know the amount of input being received from community services and how this varies both on an area of residence and practitioner basis. Box 4.3 gives a list of client groups which might be included in this category. For individuals in some or all of these groups it might be useful to record every contact. Details of what took place during the contact would not be necessary, only the fact that a contact has taken place. Additional information about the nature of the contact could be obtained by occasional surveys. It would also not be necessary to record this contact data on all the client groups all the time. Certain groups could be selected for recording one year and others in subsequent years.

Box 4.3   Client groups of particular importance

Preschool children	Homeless people
Mentally ill	Schoolchildren
Carers	Learning difficulty
Children with special needs	Travelling people
Addiction	TB
Sensory deficiency	People with accidental injury
Ethnic minorities	Terminally ill
Vulnerable families	Single parents
Young physically disabled, e.g. multiple sclerosis, head injury, incontinence	
Elderly people, e.g. frail, specific disability	
Residents of residential and nursing homes	

A simple monthly hand tally by each community nurse would suffice for recording at levels 1 and 2. A mark would be made in each relevant category for each visit or session and these would be added up, say, on a weekly basis and submitted possibly monthly or even 3 or 6 monthly. The information obtained from these hand tallies would be used for two purposes:

1. to obtain a clear picture of the type of service which is being delivered and to which client groups;
2. as a starting point for occasional in-depth 'ad hoc' surveys relating to patients in particular client groups and diagnostic categories and for analysis of process measures (e.g. outcomes) such as sources of referral, waiting times for a particular service, etc.

The fact that the information is being used in these ways should help to ensure that it is recorded with reasonable accuracy.

Level 3: detailed person-based records

Finally, there are certain patients with complex ongoing health-care needs for whom it is important to have a patient-based record analogous to the hospital discharge record to ensure that health (and social) care needs can be identified, to monitor the adequacy of service provision and ensure that as many individuals as possible are offered any necessary screening, preventive and other services. Sometimes a patient-based record is needed in order to achieve linkage between hospital and community record systems so that patients with conditions of particular interest or importance can be followed up after discharge from hospital.

There are also specific client groups where it is important to be able to monitor the progress of individuals through the health (and social) care system: for example, preschool children, people with specific physical disabilities (e.g. multiple sclerosis, Parkinson's disease, head injury, epilepsy), people with learning difficulties, carers and people with infections such as HIV and tuberculosis. Such records are well established for preschool children and those who suffer from tuberculosis but have not generally been developed for surveillance of patients with other conditions. The kind of information required for these client groups would include numbers and prevalence rates for different age and sex categories; number of people in the subgroups, in age and sex groupings; health in terms of functional status, met and unmet needs; social care needs, including equipment, services, financial and other support; quantification of health service input to the subgroup; assessment of the health gain achieved by the various inputs and whether resources are being deployed to the best possible effect. Baseline information would be recorded on a single occasion with updating being requested at intervals (probably not more frequently than annually).

OTHER SOURCES OF INFORMATION ON HEALTH AND SOCIAL CARE NEEDS

We have shown that by aggregating data recorded about individuals, community nurses can obtain detailed information about a wide variety of population subgroups. However, it will often be necessary to supplement this information from other sources. Community nurses themselves may conduct their own special surveys and considerably more use should be made of this type of activity. For example, information routinely recorded about breast feeding or smoking could be used to create sampling frames for further in-depth investigations or for evaluating interventions. Other routine data sources should also be exploited and the subjective view of professionals and consumers sought.

Examples of routine data sources include mortality rates (all-cause and for specific causes), hospital discharge rates (also all-cause and for specific causes and for both general and psychiatric hospitals), referral rates to hospitals by general practitioners, cancer incidence rates, breast and cervical screening uptake and a wide variety of information relating to births. This information may be obtained from sources such as the Registrar General (Scotland) or the Office of Population Censuses and Surveys in England, from hospital discharge records, from cancer registers and from other health authority information systems.

Professionals (for example, general practitioners, hospital doctors, community nurses, social workers, occupational therapists and physiotherapists) provide an important perspective. In addition, the views of particular client and diagnostic groups may also be sought, either directly or through relevant voluntary organisations and self-help groups. Focus groups are increasingly being used in this respect. Other organisations such as Citizens Advice Bureaux may also be able to provide information about health and health needs. Finally, surveys may be commissioned to obtain information for the population in general or for specific groups.

In addition, the potential exists for community nurses to take a lead role in recording and analysis of morbidity data in primary care. Although an increasing number of general practitioners now record morbidity for all their patients, the majority record only those conditions which attract special payments (asthma or diabetes). If, as suggested above, community nurses were to develop patient-based records for all those individuals with complex and long-term health and social care needs, then these in aggregate would provide not only a morbidity index for a wide variety of medical conditions but also detailed information about the health and social care needs of people with these conditions and for a wide variety of other population subgroups such as those listed in Box 4.3. This would be an enormously powerful tool, enabling community nurses and others to focus on very specific issues such as the needs of people with learning difficulties and associated epilepsy; or of younger people with Parkinson's disease; or women suffering postnatal depression or anxiety.

EVALUATION BY PUBLIC HEALTH NURSES: OUTCOMES AND OTHER MEASURES

It is impossible to measure the value of community nursing by the traditional methods for recording and analysing community nursing activity. More sensitive methods are required which focus on process and outcomes rather than quantifying tasks and activity. Because many community services are inadequately evaluated, it is particularly important to be able to derive information about the outcomes of health service interventions. Indicators might include: hospital utilisation rates (admission rates and lengths of stay); accident rates in children and older people; the outcome of rehabilitation measures; the care of people with particular health conditions (e.g. rheumatoid arthritis, long-term neurological problems), the care of elderly people and younger physically disabled people living in residential and nursing homes; patient satisfaction; immunisation uptake; breast-feeding rates; uptake of cervical, breast and other screening activities; waiting times for provision of aids and adaptations. Examples of suitable methods for presenting this type of data might include:

- annual reports on the health status of and adequacy of support for specific client groups, such as younger physically disabled people, single-parent families, homeless families, travelling people, people with specific disabilities;

- evaluations of specific interventions: for example, for smoking cessation, diet modification, encouraging exercise and breast feeding, accident prevention, reducing the prescription of hypnotics and other central nervous system drugs, encouraging residual 'defaulters' to accept screening and immunisation;
- annual reports on the health status and adequacy of health service input for communities or localities and general practices;
- monitoring the proportion of terminally ill people who are cared for satisfactorily in their own homes.

These reports would be presented for initial review by colleagues and subsequently by members of other professions and organisations. They would provide a basis for lively debate, thus stimulating the spread of good practice and helping to formulate future plans.

THE IMPORTANCE OF FEEDBACK

Community nurses should move from a position in which they record information about their own activities as a means of justifying their own work to one in which they provide information about the health and health-care needs and value of health-care interventions for defined populations and population subgroups. There should also be a shift in emphasis from only recording data towards more meaningful analysis and lively scrutiny by community nurses themselves. Community nurses should become principal users of their own data; they should not accept the role of passive collectors of data for use by others.

It is well recognised that those responsible for providing data will do so accurately and completely only if it is clear to them that good use is being made of the data. This means that community nurses – as data providers – must have regular and timely feedback of analysis from their data for scrutiny and interpretation. Even this would be a major step forward but community nurses should aim to establish a much more proactive role in managing and developing their information systems. At the very least, community nurses should have access to facilities for ad hoc analyses of their data and should contribute to the selection of populations and groups for more in-depth recording or special surveys. However, there is little reason why community nurses should not take the lead in developing information systems and ensuring that all information recorded is used to maximum effect. This role would require a great deal of vision and imagination with a clear focus on public health, in particular finding out more about and working to improve the health of the population.

Justification of the role of community nursing would have no part in such a development; the central role of this workforce in improving public health would soon be self-evident. Likewise, technological considerations, such as computer hardware and software, should not play an important role; these are commonplace tools of the trade and should be very much subservient rather than leading development.

CONCLUSION

Community nurses are uniquely able to forge alliances with the many health service and social work professionals, voluntary organisations and self-help groups which are in a position to improve the lot of elderly people, those with long-term disabilities, family carers, homeless people and other vulnerable groups. It is their responsibility to identify in a defined population, such as a general practice or locality, those individuals who have health and social care needs and to do what they can to assemble the resources required to meet these needs. This can be achieved both for individuals and, by advocacy, for client groups. A central role for community nurses in carrying out public health activity is to use the information they have to hand to design services that meet the identified needs of the population groups.

Any data collection system is time consuming and therefore data collected should be used to improve services and not merely to satisfy historical needs of outdated management systems. The amount of data collected should relate to the complexity of clients' needs and to the likely duration of their need for intervention. A three-tier system was proposed in this chapter which would allow flexibility in recording systems and prevent unnecessary data being collected.

Community nurses have the potential to take the lead in developing information systems and ensuring that all information recorded is used to maximum effect. We owe it to those who need this care to provide the leadership necessary to release the energies, knowledge and skills of the community nurse workforce to achieve these crucial objectives.

REFERENCES

Cowan R 1840 Vital statistics of Glasgow illustrating the sanitary condition of the population. Paper read before the statistical section of the British Association, 21 September
Down Lisburn Trust 1994 Integrated health and social care in Down Lisburn Trust, Northern Ireland. Down Lisburn Health and Social Census Trust, Linenhall Street, Lisburn, Co Antrim, BT28 1LU
Perry R C 1844 Facts and observations on the sanitary state of Glasgow during the last year showing the connection existing between poverty, disease and crime with appendices containing reports from the district surgeons. Pamphlet dedicated to the Lord Provost of Glasgow
Womersley J 1987 The evolution of health information services. In: McLachlan G (ed) Improving the common weal: aspects of Scottish health services 1900–1984. Nuffield Provincial Hospitals Trust, London

FURTHER READING

Lockhart K, Womersley J, Black D 1992 Community nursing in Glasgow: a vision for the future. Greater Glasgow Health Board, Glasgow
McIntosh H, Womersley J 1986 Children with spina bifida: the role of the health visitor in tertiary prevention. Health Visitor 59: 380–382
Roberts C et al 1996 The proof of the pudding … Health Service Journal, 106(5494): 27
Stone D 1996 Visiting time. Health Service Journal 11th April: 28–29

5

Introducing the social model of health

Rosie Ilett   Kate Munro

INTRODUCTION

The theory and practice of medicine and popular notions of health are dominated by medical models, concerned largely with symptoms of illness and treatment. This paradigm developed historically through increasingly scientific approaches to healing and caring, underpinned by observations of malfunction and disease. The widespread adoption of this model has inhibited both the discussion of the reasons for ill health and the initiation and introduction of services and treatments which assume a broader perspective.

This chapter will chart this process and present the social model of health and its implications for nursing practice. By looking at different groups within society, it highlights the importance of social factors in relation to health and the potential consequences of failing to take social factors into account in providing health care. The chapter also charts the increasing acceptance of a social model of health through WHO policies and nurses' particular role in facilitating social support and social networks at individual and community levels. Examples of this within both research and practice will be discussed, using domestic violence and postnatal support as case studies.

THE ONSET OF THE DISEASE MODEL

The development and dominance of the medical model of health can be traced back to the influence of the European Enlightenment on medical theory and practice. Until that point, in the 17th and 18th centuries, beliefs and understandings about the world were generally constrained by localised and individual experiences. Illness and health were conceived within religious notions of the links between humanity and God and relationships to external forces. This period marked the onset of modern science and a rejection of earlier knowledge and ideas as being subjective and not open to scrutiny.

As a way of viewing, interacting with and organising the natural world, science increasingly saw itself as objective, with professions emerging whose status was based on possessing specialist knowledge. The impetus to evolve a medical science transformed existing hospitals into places where doctors, through observing patients, became scientists and specialists. A medicine then developed which emphasised and charted differences and deviations from the norm, which could be treated and righted by practical and quantifiable interventions. The focus on disease advanced the medical model of health, as it created a synthesis and interchangeability between health and illness. Observing and treating patients, classifying and describing malfunction led to an individualising of the concepts of health and ill health (Open University 1992).

THE POWER OF DOCTORS

The increasingly rational and categorised scientific society grew in tandem with the professional power and growing expertise of doctors. Being afforded the ability to diagnose, cure and treat ill health, within a social and cultural structure which sees this as vital and essential, gives doctors an authority not to be underestimated and inevitably results in health being seen in terms of illness and disease (Kennedy 1981). This is the reverse of developing positive notions of health and well-being and gives credibility to the medical model.

Doctors have an extremely important influence on how individuals and groups experience health and health care. Working within hospital settings as specialists and community settings as general practitioners, doctors deal with people from all groups within society, presenting with all types of symptoms and feelings. Traditional roles afford doctors status as:

That little bit different from other mortals – more so than practically any other member of society … for the family doctor is expected to be part physician, part priest and part social worker, dealing with humanity when it is at its most sensitive and most fragile. (Gibson 1981, p. 3)

There may have been shifts away from this image of the doctor in the last few decades but many people still feel that the authority and knowledge of a doctor are something of value, with an associated magical or symbolic element (Roberts 1985).

Patients often feel that their interaction with the doctor has been successful only if it results in an outcome like a prescription or a referral for further tests or treatment. If this is not achieved, feelings of disappointment, rejection and not being taken seriously can arise. Groups within society who feel more marginalised, for example those who are from a different socioeconomic or racial group from the doctor, are likely to experience these feelings more strongly, possibly because they find it more difficult to feel comfortable within the consultation process.

VALUE JUDGEMENTS IN MEDICINE

Increased specialisms led to classifications of physical anomalies and illness, which developed the notion and power of medical expertise (Illich 1979). Emphasising disease and dysfunction led to Western medicine's preoccupation with treating illness as its main function. The disease model 'locates disease within the person and conceptualises the sources of disease in terms of germs, physical insult or defects in the individual's physical structure or function' (Broom 1983, p. 52).

This allows choices to be made about what illness is and who is classed as being ill. Decisions on what constitutes disease are influenced by social, cultural and moral forces, which have many repercussions. Classifying a condition as a disease implies the need to find a cure, fund research, obtain resources for medical care, develop health promotional and preventive action, discover and agree symptoms and a pathology, as well as having legal and social implications (Reznek 1987).

Involving morality in defining health and illness can introduce prejudice and bigotry, with groups within the population being marginalised and blamed for their own condition (Kennedy 1981). In 19th-century Britain, for example, the fear of sexuality meant that masturbation was seen as a grave illness, treatable by bromide, surgery or incarceration in a mental institution. People with HIV are a more recent example of a group viewed as either responsible or not responsible for their own condition. Although HIV infection itself is greeted with public sympathy, the inferred mode of infection determines at what level. Heterosexual women, haemophiliacs or children are seen as innocent and undeserving of HIV infection while gay men or injecting drug users may be seen as guilty. This approach, as many observers have pointed out, leads to differences in funding for services and research, education and information giving and in the way that people act individually and collectively (Patton 1990).

Some conditions can then be focused on at the expense of others, with the medical profession encouraging the classification of diseases in a certain way. Concepts of good and bad diseases and illnesses develop, crucial in terms of public and political perceptions and in relation to limited resources.

Examinations of public perceptions of illness, like the Oregon experiment, show how this can operate. In this scheme, begun in 1994, the US state of Oregon extended health care to those with no medical insurance, who would otherwise receive no free services bar emergency treatment. Medical professionals devised priorities, modified after public consultation, which formed the basis of resource allocation. Diseases seen as self-induced were rated as less deserving of treatment than those where the individual was seen to have behaved responsibly. For example, a patient needing a liver transplant through alcohol-induced cirrhosis would be ignored, while a teetotal patient with equivalent needs would be treated (McRae 1994). A hierarchy of disease and conditions, clearly subjective and not value-free, is then created.

EXCLUSIONS FROM HEALTH AND HEALTH CARE

Moral frameworks around decision making about health and health care can lead to exclusion and to some groups being denied equity. The tendency to focus on lifestyles as a primary cause of disease, for example, leads to attempts to encourage people to change behaviour to avoid possible ill health. Blaming individuals for their continued participation in unhealthy activities, like smoking and drinking, inevitably results. Recent coverage of doctors being reluctant to allocate services to overweight people, the unemployed and people with no dependants demonstrates this potential. Services are then not offered to those entitled to them but only to those judged worthy of receipt (Rogers 1994). For example, this can lead to attempts to tackle smoking in pregnancy through providing factual information about the dangers but with no connection made with the contradictory reasons why women continue to smoke and in what social and economic context this may be taking place.

Therefore, the medical model ignores social inequalities and differences which can affect an individual's health and well-being for many complex and interrelated reasons. It allows the exclusion of groups of people from the mainstream and gives them less power. Being black in a racist society, being long-term unemployed, being a single parent or a woman experiencing discrimination impacts both directly and indirectly and can cause detrimental effects on health. If these connections are denied, pathologies and stereotypes can grow which are antipathetic to full involvement in society, including access to health care and the ability to obtain relief.

Women

The medical model of health has disenfranchised and stereotyped a number of groups within society, the classic example being women. The theory and practice of medicine relating to women has traditionally been concerned with biological function and dysfunction, with women's complex reproductive systems and ability to bear children differentiating them from men in their collective and individual experiences of health and health care. Women have been viewed within a model relating to bodily functions, not a social model which conceptualises women within a wider context (Glasgow Healthy City Project 1996).

The construction of women's health based on childbirth still forms the basis of medical management of women and the training of staff who work with women, like nurses, health visitors, midwives, gynaecologists, obstetricians and general practitioners (Reid 1982, Broom 1983). The ability to reproduce, within a sanctioned heterosexual family relationship, dominates most women's experience of health and health care. Pregnancy is a natural part of most women's lives yet for many women, it is organised and monitored on medical lines. This definition of pregnancy contrasts with the notions that women receive about childbearing. Girls assimilate views that pregnancy does not equal illness yet on becoming pregnant, women are often stunned that it is treated as such by medical staff (Miles 1991).

As well as pregnancy and childbirth becoming increasingly medicalised, the onset of the menopause, which removes that possibility, is an important focus for the evolution of new medical treatments and procedures. As recently as 1979 it was felt that 'the medical profession has traditionally taken very little interest in the menopause' (Bristol Women's Studies Group 1979, p. 100). Since then there has been widespread development and prescribing of hormone replacement therapy. However, some critics have seen this as an attempt to make medication acceptable through appealing to women's concerns about their physical appearance and sexual performance and by constructing a pathology about women's hormones (Anderson 1983, Worcester & Whatley 1992).

As well as taking on the role of patients and recipients of health care, women have always been part of the caring process but with unequal access to power or decision making. The onset of the modern health service occurred after the suppression of women's lay medicine, when women's entry to education and the professions was restricted. The status of medicine was fairly low and was raised partly through developing a male-defined vocation. Women, it was feared, would soften the profession and its new-found intellectual and scientific image (Blake 1990).

The increased authority of the male medical profession paralleled the marginalisation of women as practitioners and healers. Many have documented the historical importance of wise women in undertaking lay diagnoses and using natural treatments, noting the empirical basis of many of the old wives tales that grew from their experiments (Ehrenreich & English 1977, Chamberlain 1980, Hekman 1990, Miles 1991, Kramarae & Treichler 1992, Bone 1994). Midwifery descends directly from this activity as wise women tended to pregnancies and births. Many feel that the murders of women as witches between the 14th and 17th centuries were provoked by a desire to obliterate the knowledge and independence of women and to diminish women by stereotyping them as prey to uncontrollable emotions and sexual desires (Ehrenreich & English 1977, Kramarae & Treichler 1992, Turner 1995).

Lesbians

Women have been regarded within society and in areas like medicine and health care as having different sexual needs and desires from men. This relates to the contradictory, yet interchangeable, images of women as mothers and bearers of children and also as uncontrollably sexual creatures – the 'virgin and whore' archetypes.

Women's sexuality and sexual expression have been the subject of much social and political control throughout history. In line with the medical model of health and dominant social models which define women in terms of childbearing potential and relationships to men, women who deviate from the norm tend to be excluded from equal access to services and society. Women who choose to remain childless, women whose children have different fathers, women who are lone parents, women who have children past the acceptable age range – all fail to conform to the accepted mores that determine women's behaviour and social responsibilities in relation to childbirth. For women who choose not to have sex with men and have sex instead with women or who identify women as their preferred life companions, there is even more likelihood of discrimination.

Over the last few years in Britain, following work in the United States, there has been a rising awareness of the health and health needs of lesbians and women who have sex with women. There have been increasing demands from lesbians for a recognition that the different life experiences of lesbians, particularly in relation to living in a society which prefers and promotes heterosexuality, affect health, whether emotional, mental or physical. Many feel that social pressure prevents lesbians from obtaining equal access to health care, due to prejudice that may be experienced if women are 'out' about their sexual preferences to health workers, alongside widespread assumptions that everyone is heterosexual, which can affect diagnoses and options within consultations.

The lack of research and correct public health information about lesbian health can contribute to the onset of illness. For example, fewer lesbians than heterosexual women have cervical smear tests or breast screening, yet the limited research available shows that lesbians are at higher than average risk for some types of cancers and so should be taking up screening. This is not because cancer attacks a woman because she is a lesbian but because of a range of predisposing factors to which lesbians might be susceptible (McClure & Vespry 1994). For example, these could include a tendency to drink and smoke more than heterosexual women, which may relate to pubs and clubs often playing an important social role as a meeting-place and safe environment for lesbians or to use of alcohol or cigarettes as supports in a homophobic society.

Black and ethnic minority communities

People from black and ethnic minority communities experience health and health care differently from the majority white population in the United Kingdom. As black and ethnic minority communities are not a homogeneous group, it is difficult to generalise and the lack of health data or statistics classified by ethnic origin makes comment more difficult. However, facts that clearly impact on health include:

- unemployment amongst black and ethnic minorities, particularly for women and young people, is at least twice that of white counterparts;
- the overall income for ethnic minority households is less than the average for white households and supports more people;
- people from black and ethnic minorities are more likely to live in poor housing in inner-city areas (Avan & Brown 1994).

Medical indicators also point to differences in health status. For example, people of Indian origin have higher mortality rates from heart disease than average and nearly twice as many babies of Pakistan-born mothers die before their first birthday than those of other UK mothers (Laughlin & Black 1995).

As with lesbians and other groups, other issues lie behind some of the morbidity and mortality figures and the patterns of health-seeking and health-endangering behaviour which form traditional views of health. In particular, social and economic factors affect health and many researchers link the apparent disposition of some black and ethnic minority groups to certain clinical disorders directly with exclusion and disadvantage. For example, although African-Caribbean women are prone to hypertension, cerebrovascular diseases and strokes and may have a genetic propensity, many live in poverty, work in low-paid stressful jobs and suffer the double discrimination of racism and sexism (Douglas 1994). The constant experiences of poverty, unemployment, poor housing, racism and discrimination undergone by people from black and ethnic minority communities in the UK may also directly affect mental health. This may be the explanation for what appears to be proportionally higher rates of mental illness than within the white population (Littlewood & Lipsedge 1982).

Many people from black and ethnic minority communities are excluded from full involvement in making health choices by the lack of health education and health information materials in minority languages and difficulties in accessing health care because of language barriers. As with women overall and lesbians, people from black and ethnic minority communities can experience discrimination from the wider society and from staff within health and social care settings. Racism clearly affects life choices and health, whether physical, emotional or mental in expression.

People living in poverty

A medical model of health is concerned with individual pathologies and explanations of illness and disease. Yet recognising large-scale patterns of difference means that inequalities in health caused by socioeconomic factors such as poverty have to be understood. The links between people living in poverty and ill health were a focus of much of the work done by early public health campaigners in the 19th century. They emphasised the connections between environmental and social conditions and the health of the population and advocated widespread change to improve health.

Looking at figures relating to poverty and health clarifies the relationship. Standard measurements of life expectancy, for example, show that a child born into social class V (the least privileged group within the population, comprising people working as labourers and cleaners, according to the Registrar General's classification) is likely to die 8 years earlier than a child of parents in social class I (the richest group, of people working as doctors and lawyers). Children and adults are likely to be more frequently ill the lower down the Registrar General's scale they are, with a parallel correlation between adults defining their own health as poor and their socioeconomic status (Laughlin & Black 1995).

People living in poverty are more likely to spend more time in the home, which in turn is more likely to be substandard and hard to heat, and to spend a higher proportion of their income on heating their homes than the average. Limited income means that each day choices have to be made which have health implications, like choosing between buying food or putting money into the gas meter, for example. Research shows that people on low incomes spend more proportionately on household items, food, heating and lighting than better-off people yet often receive or have access to services and goods which are inferior or more expensive (Fyfe 1994). A House of Commons official report of 1993 found that many elderly people were so frightened of incurring debt that they resorted to living in the cold. This was similar to the findings of a 1992 Age Concern survey, which found that the room temperatures in most elderly people's homes was below World Health Organisation guidelines (Sheldrick 1994).

Living in such circumstances, with less access to work (which brings income as well as the support and self-worth that many find through their job), affects quality of life and health on more than just a physical level. There has been increased recognition of the stress and anxiety experienced by many people living in poverty, which also directly affect physical health.

Yet, as with other groups discussed in this chapter, these factors may not be recognised by medical staff, who may only be able to respond to the immediate presenting situation. The inability to provide appropriate resources may also inhibit more suitable responses being suggested. As one writer comments:

There is some evidence that people living in the most deprived areas experience services which are poorer in quality. Lower social class patients have been found to be less likely to receive specialist referrals and to receive less information voluntarily from GPs. (Curtice 1994, p. 77)

People with disabilities

The experience of disabled people in accessing health and health care differs from the other groups discussed, as generally disabled people receive more care and assistance because of their disability or condition than the average. Throughout Western society, disabled people have been seen by medical discourse as being different, impaired and outside the norm and therefore in need of health and social care (Abberley 1993, Harrison 1993). Medical and social responses have been developed to provide help and assistance, which have tended to operate outside mainstream society. The recent changes in community care have partly reframed this approach but many disabled people are obliged to depend on others, with little chance to make autonomous life choices, due to the prevalence of the medical model.

For many disabled people born in the UK before the 1950s, there was no option to being put into an institution. One woman, born in 1946, whose cerebral palsy inhibited her speaking or walking, failed an intelligence test at 5 years and was classified by doctors as an 'imbecile'. Regarded as unfit for education, she was admitted to a large institution for mentally handicapped people, where she remained for many years (Humphries & Gordon 1992).

The development of the disability rights movement over the last 20 years in the UK and the USA has exposed much of the treatment meted out to disabled people, whether with a mental, physical or sensory impairment, and many of the attitudes that have made it possible. The medicalisation of disabled people has caused a separation and schism in relation to wider society, with disabled people being presented with a social role determined by the nature of their impairment and their seeming inability to contribute fully. The sickness/dependent role is often the only one offered and as some writers comment, the power of the medical profession to define and decide who is classified as ill or sick or in need of help is particularly pertinent to people who are disabled (Oliver 1993).

The life experience of a disabled person can be decided by the way that medical staff explain and interpret the individual impairment to those involved at the birth and the choices that then start to be made on the basis of those, often off the cuff, remarks. Lack of information and support can cause numerous problems, as an account from Margaret Bennett, born in 1925 with cerebral palsy, reveals:

If any child was born physically handicapped it was hushed up and kept out of the way. In my family my disability was just ignored. Mum and dad didn't tell me that I was disabled or why or anything. When I was quite little I asked my dad if the doctors had said anything when I was born, whether they had said I was different from other children. My dad just told me that I had a bit of rheumatism. (quoted in Humphries & Gordon 1992, p. 27)

DECONSTRUCTING THE MEDICAL MODEL OF HEALTH AND PRESENTING AN ALTERNATIVE – THE SOCIAL MODEL OF HEALTH

The focus on disease and the need to restore normality by treatments advanced the medical model of health. The medical model sees health as being about illness and ill health determined by the individual patient. It is a negative concept, focusing on biological determinism, with many failings in interpreting the human condition. It does not easily accommodate the differing experiences of people, involved in numerous interactions and subject to many influences – some voluntary and some not – which can affect their health. It is basically a reductionist process, where people are seen as collections of parts, not as a holistic whole (Kennedy 1981).

From its inception the medical model has been challenged as being inadequate in explaining the complexities of health and illness. Many have proposed a social model of health which views health as positive, not negative, involving all of society, not just the individual patient. The 19th-century philanthropism, where the middle classes worked to educate poor people about hygiene and diet, developed much of the awareness that health was determined by issues like sanitation and poverty. Social and cultural changes and wider understandings around gender, race, sexuality and disability have allowed more extensive criticisms to be made of the medical model.

The World Health Organisation's well-known constitutional definition has formed the cornerstone of much of this work, where 'health is a state of complete physical, mental and social well-being, and not merely the absence of disease or infirmity' (WHO 1946). This proposes a health model explicitly informed by knowledge about social interactions, with 'the importance of socioeconomic factors and their interaction with people's lifestyles in determining both quality of life and cause of death' being taken fully into account (Burns 1994).

The social model of health has been seen by groups such as women, disabled people, community activists and lesbians and gay men as providing an explanation of how society creates health and ill health and how factors such as discrimination and bias operate to exclude full participation and affect health. The social model's deconstruction of the medical model and medical notions and discourse can help reveal how differences between individuals and groups of people can lead to prejudice. It allows the expansion of a vision of health and links in with wider social and cultural change to achieve social equality, alongside health equality.

DEVELOPING A WHO HEALTH-PROMOTING STRATEGY: ALMA-ATA TO OTTAWA

Much of the shift in conceptualising health has occurred since the 1970s. Changes partly initiated through the WHO have encouraged governments, statutory and voluntary bodies who provide health care and other services to work together to improve public health. Until then, the WHO concentrated on a medical model of health, with 'an optimal disease-free state' being the overall objective (Jones & Meleis 1993, p. 1). A main concern was the eradication of disease in developing countries, through the transfer of expert skills from the industrialised world (Davies & Kelly 1993). Since then, connections between the environment, social, cultural and economic issues and the health of populations worldwide have begun to be made. This new paradigm has led to radical approaches being taken to public health, encompassing concepts previously not seen as relative to medicine and health care.

One catalyst for this change was the 1978 WHO International Conference and Declaration on Primary Health Care, held in Alma-Ata in the Soviet Union. This assembly initiated the worldwide strategy of Health for All by the Year 2000, which argued that countries are responsible for the health of their population and need to set diverse health targets, achievable through genuine strategic approaches (Kelly & Charlton 1995). These require the cooperation of a wide range of organisations and embrace notions of health promotion through community empowerment, participation and self-determination. The inclusion of these methods gave the opportunity to consider and challenge the insidious effects of discrimination and social inequality on collective and individual health and well-being. It also meant that widening the definitions of health led to the need to develop more imaginative resources and services and to develop a different set of health indicators and measures.

After the seeds of change were sown in Alma-Ata, the WHO continued the expansion of its health agenda at Ottawa at the First International Conference on Health Promotion, in 1986. This happened in the light of discussions post Alma-Ata, which led to the birth of a ground-breaking WHO definition of health promotion and a desire to define and set its principles and parameters at the Ottawa Conference (Davies & Kelly 1993, O'Neill 1993). This new model of health promotion drew on many ideas of the grassroots movements and campaigns of the 1960s and 1970s which advocated community participation and local action and the rights of individual citizens within wider society (Ashton 1992, O'Brien 1995). In the intervening years since Alma-Ata the development of proposals to promote collaborative health-promoting work led to the launch in 1986 of the worldwide Healthy City Project. This programme:

Using community participation as a method ... seeks to reduce inequalities, strengthen health gain, and reduce morbidity and mortality ... its method and philosophy mark a decisive shift in ways of thinking about health in an urban environment. (Davies & Kelly 1993, p. 3)

Cities in the UK, like Glasgow, Liverpool, Belfast and Camden, London, given Healthy City status due to inequalities in health and major social and economic problems, have since then been working on interagency policy making, service planning and delivery in a concerted attempt to promote positive health. These activities have already yielded exciting results, in terms of a wider recognition of the benefits of multiagency working, the evolution of new types of services tailored to fit the needs of geographic communities and groups within them and an increasing acceptance of what health is and who is involved in it.

The new public health movement

These moves within the WHO fed into and drew on work happening throughout Europe and beyond. This type of activity has become known as the new public health movement (reflecting its close ideological links to the pioneering public health movement in the 19th century) and specifically makes links between external circumstances and individual and communal health. The social model is central to the theories of this movement, which 'identifies environment and lifestyle as key mediators in the relationship between structural position and health experience and classifies both as potential areas for interventions' (Davison & Smith, 1995, p. 92). This means that communities are encouraged to develop their own collective responses to unhealthy situations, which may be campaigning and challenging, alongside recognising that individuals may need personalised support and services to overcome some of the external issues affecting them.

This work has been most concretely expressed through some of the WHO Healthy City Project initiatives, where strategic approaches have been taken to wider social and health changes, with the support of funders and service providers. Running parallel to this, services seen as important by communities, empowered to determine their own health, have been developed. For example, Glasgow has developed city-wide health strategies and policies linking in with and supporting locally based projects and services, including complementary therapy centres, women's health services, men's health work, antipoverty initiatives and lay health worker schemes.

INFLUENCE OF THE SOCIAL MODEL OF HEALTH ON NURSING INTERVENTIONS

Despite the growing influence of the social model on our understanding of health, it appears to have had a limited impact on the ways in which health care is organised and delivered. The *Health of the Nation* White Paper (DoH 1995) noted that 'Despite the considerable attention paid to the associations between a range of factors and ill health there is little practical guidance available on effective interventions in the health arena to address health variations'. A further report (DoH 1996) found that while it is likely that differential exposure to health-damaging or health-promoting physical and social environments is the main explanation for observed variations in health, the evidence on practical public health interventions which might reduce health variations is weak. As a result, work on variations in health remains undervalued and marginalised with little systematic activity on the design and implementation of effective measures taking place within the NHS.

This creates a significant tension for health professionals working in both hospital and community settings. In order to encourage the development of social interventions which promote health, organisational commitment by way of research, policy directives, support, resources, training and alliances will be necessary. However, while nurses have been challenged on how little of current nursing activity is consistent with the WHO definition (Chinn 1987) and urged to consider constraining social factors which limit their clients' achievement of health (Meleis 1990), the lack of research into and policy guidance on social model interventions has created confusion about the practical measures which should be implemented.

Although largely unsupported by policy developments, there is a growing body of practice-based evidence for nursing interventions based on a social model where factors such as social support, integration and isolation have been addressed in order to increase health status. For example, interventions in domestic violence and in postnatal support and the implications for health care in each have been described in both research and in case studies of good practice.

Domestic violence is a health service issue

Recent public education and awareness-raising campaigns, most notably the Zero Tolerance Campaign, have sought to overcome the historical secrecy, guilt and denial which have surrounded domestic violence. However, this is an area which has received little systematic attention or research in terms of either provision, protection or prevention. As a result, knowledge about the extent and nature of domestic violence is patchy but is developing as methods of calculating prevalence improve and women's own accounts of their experiences of abuse are acknowledged.

Domestic violence is not a recorded crime and so difficult to quantify but one survey of police records (Dobash & Dobash 1979) found that violence towards a female partner accounted for 25% of all reported assaults. A review of the 1992 British Crime Survey, which includes interviews with the public as well as official records, found that 11% of women reported physical violence against them in their relationship (Mirrlees-Black 1995), while a study in North London found that 27% of women had experienced physical violence at some point in their lives, 37% experienced mental cruelty and 23% had been raped (Mooney 1993). However, despite the growing body of research evidence, domestic violence continues to be secretive and hidden. In 1993 the House of Commons Home Affairs Committee reported that 'the extent of the problem … is perhaps only now beginning to be properly revealed' and in the United States the FBI believes that domestic violence is the most unreported crime. They estimate that it may be 10 times more unreported than rape.

Domestic violence takes many forms. It is defined by the Home Affairs Committee on Domestic Violence (Parliamentary Select Committee on Violence in Marriage 1979) as including 'any form of physical, sexual or emotional abuse which takes place within the context of a close relationship'. Domestic violence is distinct from other forms of intrafamilial violence such as elder abuse or violence against men by women because of its roots in society's beliefs about the way in which power and control should be exercised within families and in the traditional ideas of the man as the dominant, proprietorial head of the house. For many women, domestic violence includes physical, sexual and emotional abuse which can range from minor assaults to permanent injury or death. The implications of domestic violence for the NHS are considerable. Victims of abuse are more likely to have poor health, chronic pain problems, depressions, addictions, problem pregnancies and to have attempted suicide (Jaffe et al 1986, Amaro et al 1990, Stark & Flitcraft 1991, Plichta 1992, Mooney 1993). Psychosocial problems such as panic attacks, depression and high anxiety occur more frequently amongst women who have experienced domestic violence (Walker 1979) and it has been suggested that there is an association with delayed physical effects such as arthritis, heart disease and hypertension (Council on Scientific Affairs 1992). Furthermore, the health service is likely to be the first formal agency to which women turn for help. Research undertaken with women who had escaped violent relationships found that 80% had sought medical attention at least once while 40% sought it on at least five occasions. In contrast, only 2% had reported a violent attack to the police (Dobash & Dobash 1979).

This gives the health service a unique opportunity and responsibility to intervene but despite this, health professionals often fail to identify a large proportion of the women consulting them who are experiencing domestic violence (Borkowski et al 1983, Pahl 1985). Consequently, many victims of violence pass through the current system undetected. Studies have shown that women who had experienced domestic violence were generally dissatisfied with the response they received from health services (McWilliams & McKiernan 1993, Tayside Women and Violence Working Group 1994) and one study indicated that they rated health professionals lower than solicitors, social workers, police and clergy in terms of their effectiveness (McWilliams & McKiernan 1993).

A common response to women experiencing abuse is the prescription of tranquillisers (Tayside Women and Violence Working Group 1994). This may help the woman cope with some aspects of her situation but may also make her more vulnerable to assault through numbing her alertness to the dangers she faces. Victims of domestic violence have been shown to be 14 times more likely to attempt suicide than non-abused women (Amaro et al 1990) and so a prescription for tranquillisers or painkillers in such cases may serve to further increase this risk. Health professionals may find it easier to prescribe medication than to raise the issue of domestic violence but there are clear limitations to a medical model intervention in which only the health effects of violence, whether physical or emotional, are diagnosed and treated. A social model intervention would require that domestic violence is diagnosed and the service's response is based on the woman's perception of danger and her options for change in addition to the presenting somatic and mental health issues.

Early recognition of violence as the underlying cause of health problems is an important first step in identifying and appropriately treating victims and can lead to the prevention of further violence and ill health. Domestic violence is rarely an isolated event and when violence is not diagnosed it is most likely to continue and even escalate (Andrews & Brown 1988). Routine identification would be consistent with an approach based on the medical ethical principle of beneficence which places a duty on health-care staff to address the underlying cause of physical injury and disease (Council on Ethical and Judicial Affairs 1992). Identification increases the chance of intervention before it reaches a life-threatening level. The perception by women that domestic violence is life-threatening is confirmed by statistics which indicate the high risk of death. Research indicates that in 1992 40–45% of female homicide victims in England and Wales had been killed by their former or current partner, compared to 6% of male homicide victims (Mirrlees-Black 1995). The ethical principle of non-maleficence – to do no harm – also directs health professionals to address the underlying violence. If violence is missed then the treatments prescribed are likely to be inappropriate, contraindicated or even harmful. Once abuse is recognised then a number of interventions are possible but failure to acknowledge it may further a woman's sense of entrapment and self-blame and hence increase her health risks.

However, despite the risks, the possibility of domestic violence is rarely raised directly with patients and it has been estimated that only 25% of women seeking medical help will reveal that they have been abused (Dobash & Dobash 1979). Instead, many will use a 'calling card', presenting with an apparently unimportant physical symptom, and seek help indirectly. Women's reluctance to name the violence they have experienced should not be interpreted as acceptance of or collusion with the abuse. Their disclosure of abuse can be seen as courageous given the stigma that is attached, the fear of reprisals, the increased risk associated with separation from a violent partner and the belief, often reinforced by their partner, that they won't be believed or will be blamed (Pahl 1985, McWilliams & McKiernan 1993, Tayside Women and Violence Working Group 1994). In the past, health professionals may have felt unable to intervene because of a lack of confidence in their skills and because of a shared sense of helplessness in the face of society's indifference and ambivalence towards violence in the home (Heath 1992). However, by ignoring the 'calling card', health professionals not only miss the opportunity to prevent further instances of abuse but are also colluding with the continuing concealment of domestic violence.

The Scottish Needs Assessment Programme (1997) report on domestic violence proposes that it may be possible to learn from other systems such as 'CAGE' questions for the use of alcohol, which indicate that it need not be difficult to approach all attendees at health-care settings in a simple, direct and effective manner. Coupled to this would be comprehensive training for all staff to give them the skills and confidence to raise the issue and pass on appropriate information to women. This is reinforced by the views of abused women who have suggested that a helpful health service response to their needs would include the following five elements (McWilliams & McKiernan 1993):

- awareness of the possibility of domestic violence;
- recognition of signs and indicators;
- raising the issue through direct, non-judgemental questions;
- time to talk to a willing listener;
- advice and information about appropriate support services.

These elements are consistent with attempts to improve the health service response to domestic violence, which have stressed the need for staff to be 'aware that domestic violence occurs and prepared to ask key questions' (McIlwaine 1989). The Home Office Report on Domestic Violence (Smith 1989) recommended a number of steps for development within the NHS.

- The development of standard protocols for identifying women who experience domestic violence.
- The development of training programmes for staff.
- Encouraging staff to liaise with and refer to other agencies.
- The development of effective data-recording systems.

Recommendations from both abused women and the Home Office point to the importance of acknowledging the abuse, providing information on options and, with consent, referring women to other sources of support, information and refuge. Although there is little evidence of any systematic attempts to introduce these recommendations in the UK, research from the United States indicates the effectiveness of introducing staff training and protocols in accident and emergency settings. In one study, this led to an increase from 6% to 30% in the detection of women experiencing domestic violence (McLeer & Anwar 1989). Recognition, acknowledgement and concern confirm the seriousness of domestic violence and can make a significant difference to women's options for living free from violence. In contrast, silence or disinterest conveys tacit approval or acceptance, so even if a woman is not ready to leave an abusive relationship or to take other action, recognition and validation of her situation are important. This is illustrated by McWilliams & McKiernan (1993), as follows:

Interviews with the medical and health professionals showed how the violence could often be minimised and not diagnosed or identified ... this is the process which results in double victimisation of the woman, once by the perpetrator and once by the system to whom she turned for help. Where women did get advice and information, they were often enabled to take the next step. In the absence of information and advice, many of the women did not know what their rights were and could not therefore effect change in their own lives.

Optimal care for the woman in an abusive relationship thus depends not only on the effective treatment of the health effects of violence but also on the willingness of health professionals to raise the issue and on their knowledge of community resources providing safety, advocacy and support. Domestic violence generates a complex set of needs for women and their children which need to be addressed through all our community institutions. The health service doesn't hold the solution but through contact with abused women it has a key role in empowering them to begin to take steps which will change their lives.

Overcoming depression through social support

My strategy is to go to as many things as possible, and then out of all the people you meet, you'll find one or two who have got a baby near the age of yours who you get on with.

The above quote from a new mother shows she has instinctively understood, as many new mums do, that social support is an important factor in managing the depression which often accompanies the sudden onset of motherhood. In a society which idealises motherhood, our images of happy, coping mothers, stable, supportive family units and contented babies can be far removed from the reality of isolation, loneliness and stress which many new mothers experience.

Jebali (1991) identifies the commonly held assumptions that motherhood is comforting and fulfilling: mothers have natural instincts and emotional resilience and babies bring joy and harmony. The actual experience of many new mothers is more often that the abrupt transition to motherhood brings feelings of anxiety and isolation which May (1995) proposes can be exacerbated by a lack of extended family support and support networks. Studies have shown that despite the brave face women put on for the outside world (Foyster 1995), some symptoms of depression are common. These range from the mild feelings of the baby blues through moderate symptoms of despondency and helplessness associated with postnatal depression and for a few women there may also be the severe symptoms of acute anxiety, panic and feelings of physical illness of puerperal psychosis. In the UK it is estimated that 50–70% of new mothers will get the baby blues while 10–15% experience postnatal depression, of which a minority of 25% will go on to develop severe depression (Ballard et al 1994).

Postnatal depression is classified by the medical classification system DSM-IIIR under general psychotic depressive disorder. Some of the range of symptoms associated with it are as follows:

- Despondency
- Feelings of inadequacy
- Tearfulness
- Irritability
- Sleeplessness
- Guilt over not loving the baby enough

These symptoms are similar to other depressions which can arise at any other stage of life but postnatal depression occurs at any time in the first year of the baby's life. Postnatal depression is defined by Dalton (1989) as 'the presence of psychiatric symptoms severe enough to require medical help and occurring within 6 months of delivery, in a woman who has never previously had a psychotic illness'. However, despite the early onset of the depression there is evidence to suggest that powerful societal expectations of coping will result in many women suffering in silence and that these women may go undetected and unhelped for 18 months or more (Foyster 1995).

Untreated depression is associated with an increased risk of physical illness, poor parenting and marital problems (DHSS 1988) but despite this there are no clear guidelines for health-care staff on the professional roles, skills and competence needed to deal with depression in mothers with young children. This can lead to the problem being ignored or trivialised. A 1993 audit by Southampton Community and Mental Health Services Trust (Pitts 1995) found that health visitor intervention for postnatal depression accounted for 1.5% of families on caseloads. This contrasts with the national data which suggest that they should expect 10 times that number (DHSS 1983). Pitts goes on to suggest that health visitors should regard depressed mothers as a priority. The Royal College of General Practitioners (RCGP 1981) similarly urged an increased response to the support needs of mothers with a recommendation for GPs to organise and participate in patient–doctor groups.

There is now a considerable body of evidence to support the use of small support groups over the traditional medical model response of medication, hospitalisation or even counselling. Nevertheless, individual counselling can be effective. In one study (May 1995), health visitor intervention of 6–8 weekly counselling visits led to reported improvements in 87% of the women participating. However, counselling is generally seen as a prescribed treatment and, although preferable to medication, can still be seen as treating an individual pathology (May 1995). Research into group work approaches to reducing postnatal depression show that it is not only effective, appreciated and popular but in addition is cost effective and empowering (Eastwood et al 1995). Handford (1985) suggests that a group approach may be better than individual treatment as it allows women contact with their peers. A support group can not only reduce the feelings of depression but also relieve the feelings of isolation, loneliness and of being different that mothers report. A key factor of support groups appears to be the role women play in both receiving and, crucially, in giving support. At a time when they are feeling anxious about their nurturing skills and perhaps guilty about not coping well enough, the feelings of being valued that they receive from effectively supporting others are empowering and result in a growth in self-esteem (Eastwood et al 1995).

Similar work with women and with couples in Canada showed the vital role of self-help support groups, the opportunities they provide for mutual learning (Olson et al 1991) and that 'the treatment model most useful ... is one which encourages talking in confidence to other women experiencing the same difficulties' (Handford 1985). Some characteristics of effective groups are that they encourage the exploration of feelings (Holden 1987), they provide the opportunity for women to talk openly about insecurities (May 1995), the women feel that they are being listened to (Snaith 1989) and that they avoid pathologising mothers by calling themselves a 'mothers' support group' rather than 'postnatal depression support group' as women can be put off by the association with depressive illness (Foyster 1995).

The benefits of support groups for women who frequently report the additional stress of feeling they are alone are obvious. The contributory factors in postnatal depression can be biological, psychological or social, such as societal attitudes to childbearing and motherhood (Jebali 1993), but whatever the cause, the evidence from health professionals suggests that groups which provide ongoing support and contact with peers and professionals are effective in reducing depression (Pitts 1995) and increasing self-esteem (Eastwood et al 1995). The alternatives of referral to overloaded community psychiatric services, individual counselling or medication all have the limitations of heavy resource costs and of individualising the problem. In contrast, a social model approach of providing emotional support, confiding relationships, mutual learning opportunities and social support networks has been shown to be cost effective and valued by women, to reduce depression and foster well-being in women at a vulnerable time in their lives. The practice-based evidence from group work suggests that proactive intervention by way of early referral to support groups prevents women having to rely entirely on drug management of depression or even hospitalisation.

CONCLUSION: NURSING FOR HEALTH GAIN

Although the importance of social elements in relation to health has been less thoroughly investigated than other areas, there is a growing body of evidence which suggests that factors like social support, integration and isolation and social networks are all associated with health status. However, despite the recognition that there are a multiplicity of influences which affect health, the underpinning assumptions and ethos of health-care policy and interventions remain largely those of a medical model. This can create ambiguity for nurses who, despite their commitment to health, both in the hospital and the community, can be unsure of what health is and how to achieve it (Winstead-Fry 1980). The Variations in Health Subgroup of the Health of the Nation Working Group recognised this need for coherence and guidance. Their report for the Department of Health recommended that they must work actively with other government departments and other bodies to encourage social policies which promote health and that there was a need to systematically design and implement measures for health gain which address social factors (DoH 1996).

In examining two major public health issues, domestic violence and postnatal depression, we have seen that the available evidence supports a social rather than a medical model intervention in both cases. A critical feature of both interventions is that women play an active role in defining the problem and in finding their own solutions. Factors such as powerful social norms, traditional expectations of women's roles and the medicalisation of their experiences appear to be key in maintaining both as the cause of significant health problems and in preventing the further development of effective nursing roles, skills and social interventions. However, the findings available suggest that nurses can be effective in tackling the underlying causes of these health issues and in promoting physical and social environments which support positive health.

The challenge for nursing, as for other health professions, must be to promote change and development in the priority given to addressing social factors in health; to develop and disseminate case studies of good practice which provide clear guidelines on effective social interventions; and to seek to enhance the positive notions of nursing as a force for health rather than illness care.

REFERENCES

Abberley P 1993 Disabled people and normality. In: Swain J, Finkelstein V, French S, Oliver M (eds) Disabling barriers – enabling environments. Sage, London, ch 2.6, pp 107–116

Amaro H, Fried L, Cabral H, Zuckerman B 1990 Violence during pregnancy and substances abuse. American Journal of Public Health 80: 575

Anderson A 1983 Why women's health? In: McPherson A, Anderson A (eds) Women's problems in general practice. Oxford Medical Publications/Oxford University Press, Oxford

Andrews B, Brown G W 1988 Marital violence in the community. British Journal of Psychiatry 153: 305–312

Ashton J 1992 The origins of healthy cities. In: Ashton J (ed) Healthy cities. Open University Press, Milton Keynes, ch 1, pp 1–15

Avan G, Brown U 1994 Barriers to health: black and ethnic minority women. Unpublished paper

Ballard C G, Davis R, Cullen P C, Mohan R N, Dean C 1994 Prevalence of postnatal psychiatric morbidity in mothers and fathers. British Journal of Psychiatry 164: 782–788

Blake C 1990 The charge of the parasols – Women's entry to the medical profession. Women's Press, London

Bone J 1994 Women's weeds stem pregnancy. The Times 27 July

Borkowski M, Murch M, Walker V 1983 Marital violence: the community response. Tavistock Publications, London

Bristol Women's Studies Group 1979 Half the sky: an introduction to women's studies. Virago, London

Broom D 1983 Damned if we do – contradictions in women's health care. Allen and Unwin, Australia

Burns H 1994 Introduction. In: Hair S (ed) Glasgow's health, women count. Glasgow Healthy City Project Women's Health Working Group, Glasgow

Chamberlain M 1980 Old wives tales: their history, remedies and spells. Virago, London

Chinn P L 1987 Policy for health? Advanced Nursing Science 9: xii-xiii

Council on Ethical and Judicial Affairs 1992 Violence against women. Relevance for medical practitioners. Journal of the American Medical Association 267: 3184–3189

Council on Scientific Affairs 1992 Physicians and domestic violence. Ethical considerations. Journal of the American Medical Association 267: 3190–3193

Curtice L 1994 Health and welfare services. In: Fyfe G (ed) Poor and paying for it. HMSO/Scottish Consumer Council, Edinburgh, ch 5, pp 70–82

Dalton K 1989 Depression after chidbirth. Oxford University Press, Oxford

Davies J K, Kelly M P 1993 Healthy cities: research and practice. In: Davies J K, Kelly M P (eds) Healthy cities: research and practice. Routledge, London, ch 1, pp 1–13

Davison C, Smith G D 1995 The baby and the bath water: examining socio-cultural and free-market critiques of health promotion. In: Bunton R, Nettleton S, Burrows R (eds) The sociology of health promotion: critical analyses of consumption, lifestyle and risk. Routledge, London, ch 8, pp 92–99

DHSS 1983 Community nursing services returns 1972–1982. HMSO, London

DHSS 1988 On the state of the public health: the annual report of the Chief Medical Officer of the Department of Health and Social Security. HMSO, London

Dobash R E, Dobash R P 1979 Violence against wives. Free Press, New York

DoH 1995 The health of the nation. HMSO, London

DoH 1996 The health of the nation. Variations in health. What can the Department of Health and the NHS do? Report of the Variations Subgroup of the Chief Medical Officer's Health of the Nation Working Group. HMSO, London

Douglas J 1994 Black women and hypertension. In: Wilson M (ed) Healthy and wise: the essential health handbook for black women. Virago, London, ch 4, pp 43–61

Eastwood P, Horrocks E, Jones K 1995 Promoting peer group support with post natally depressed women. Health Visitor 68(4): 148–150

Ehrenreich B, English D 1977 Witches, midwives and nurses: a history of women healers. Writers and Readers, London.

Foyster L 1995 Supporting mothers: an inter-disciplinary approach. Health Visitor 68(4): 151–152

Fyfe G 1994 Life on a low income. In: Fyfe G (ed) Poor and paying for it. HMSO/Scottish Consumer Council, Edinburgh, ch 1, pp 70–82

Gibson R 1981 The family doctor: his life and history. Allen and Unwin, London.

Glasgow Healthy City Project Women's Health Working Group 1996 Action for women's health: making change through organisations. Glasgow Healthy City Project Women's Health Working Group, Glasgow

Handford P 1985 Post-partum depression. Canadian Nurse 1: 30–33

Harrison J 1993 Medical responsibilities to disabled people. In: Swain J, Finkelstein V, French S, Oliver M (eds) Disabling barriers – enabling environments. Sage, London, ch 4.3, pp 211–218

Heath I 1992 Domestic violence: the general practitioner's role. Royal College of General Practitioners Members Reference Book. Sabre Crown, London

Hekman S J 1990 Gender and knowledge: elements of a postmodern feminism. Policy Press, Cambridge

Holden J 1987 'She just listened'. Community Outlook July: 6–10

House of Commons Home Affairs Committee 1993 House of Commons Home Affairs Committee Report. HMSO, London

Humphries S, Gordon P 1992 Out of sight: the experience of disability, 1900–1950. Channel Four Books/Northcote House Books, Plymouth

Illich I 1979 Limits to medicine, medical nemesis: the expropriation of health. Penguin, Harmondsworth

Jaffe P, Wolfe D, Wilson S, Zak L 1986 Emotional and physical health problems of battered women. Canadian Journal of Psychiatry 31: 625

Jebali C A 1991 Working together to support women with postnatal depression. Health Visitor 64(12): 410–411

Jebali C A 1993 A feminist perspective on postnatal depression. Health Visitor 66(2): 59–60

Jones P S, Meleis A I 1993 Health is empowerment. Advanced Nursing Science 15(3): 1–4

Kelly M, Charlton B 1995 The modern and the postmodern in health promotion. In: Bunton R, Nettleton S, Burrows R (eds) The sociology of health promotion: critical analyses of consumption, lifestyle and risk. Routledge, London, ch 7, pp 78–91

Kennedy I 1981 The unmasking of medicine. Allen and Unwin, London

Kramarae C, Treichler P A 1992 Amazons, bluestockings and crones: a feminist dictionary. Pandora, London

Laughlin S, Black D 1995 Poverty and health. Public Health Alliance, Birmingham

Littlewood R, Lipsedge M 1982 Aliens and alienists: ethnic minorities and psychiatry. Pelican, Harmondsworth

May A 1995 Using exercise to tackle post-natal depression. Health Visitor 64(12): 146–147

McClure R, Vespry A 1994 Lesbian health guide. Queer Press, Canada

McIlwaine G 1989 Women victims of domestic violence. British Medical Journal 299: 995–996

McLeer S, Anwar R 1989 A study of battered women presenting in an emergency department. American Journal of Public Health 79: 65–66

McRae H 1994 Health-care rationing comes into the open. The Independent 26 May

McWilliams M, McKiernan J 1993 Bringing it out in the open: domestic violence in Northern Ireland. HMSO, Belfast

Meleis A I 1990 Being and becoming healthy: the core of nursing knowledge. Nursing Science Quarterly 3(3): 107–114

Miles D 1991 Women, health and medicine. Open University Press, Milton Keynes

Mirrlees-Black C 1995 Estimating the extent of domestic violence: findings from the 1992 BCS. Home Office Research and Planning Unit, London

Mooney J 1993 The hidden figure of domestic violence in North London. Islington Council, London

O'Brien 1995 Health and lifestyle: a critical mess? Notes on the dedifferentiation of health. In: Bunton R, Nettleton S, Burrows R (eds) The sociology of health promotion: critical analyses of consumption, lifestyle and risk. Routledge, London, ch 15, pp 191–206

Oliver M 1993 Re-defining disability: a challenge to research. In: Swain J, Finkelstein V, French S, Oliver M (eds). Disabling barriers – enabling environments. Sage, London, ch 1.7, pp 61–69

Olson M R, Cutler L A, Legault F 1991 Bittersweet: a postpartum depression support group. Canadian Journal of Public Health 82: 135–136

O'Neill M 1993 Building bridges between knowledge and action: the Canadian process of healthy communities indicators. In: Davies J K, Kelly M P (eds) Healthy cities: research and practice. Routledge, London, ch 10, pp 127–147

Open University 1992 Workbook 1: health as a contested concept. Department of Health and Social Welfare, Open University Press, Milton Keynes

Pahl J (ed) 1985 Private violence and public policy. Routledge and Kegan Paul, London

Parliamentary Select Committee on Violence in Marriage 1979 First special report for the Select Committee on Violence in Marriage. HMSO, London

Patton C 1990 What science knows: Formations of AIDS knowledge. In: Aggleton P, Davies P, Hart G (eds) AIDS: individual, cultural and policy dimensions. Falmer Press, Hampshire, ch 1, pp 1–19

Pitts F 1995 Comrades in adversity: the group approach. Health Visitor 68(4): 144–145

Plichta S 1992 The effects of woman abuse on health care utilization and health status: a literature review. Women's Health International 2: 154–163

RCGP 1981 Prevention of psychiatric disorders in general practice. Report from general practice 20. Royal College of General Practitioners, London

Reid M 1982 Helping those mothers: ante natal care in a Scottish peripheral estate. In: Glasgow Women's Studies Group (eds) Uncharted lives: extracts from Scottish women's experiences. Pressgang, Glasgow, ch 8, pp 163–181

Reznek L 1987 The nature of disease. Routledge and Kegan Paul, London

Roberts H 1985 The patient patients: women and their doctors. Pandora, London

Rogers L 1994 Doctors put fat patients at end of queue. Sunday Times 17 July

Scottish Needs Assessment Programme 1997 Domestic violence. Scottish Forum for Public Health Medicine, Glasgow

Sheldrick B 1994 Energy and fuel consumption. In: Fyfe G (ed) Poor and paying for it. HMSO/Scottish Consumer Council, Edinburgh, ch 3, pp 34–51

Smith L J F 1989 Domestic violence: an overview of the literature. Home Office Research Study No. 107. HMSO, London

Snaith R P 1989 Pregnancy-related psychiatric disorders. British Journal of Hospital Medicine 298: 223–226

Stark E, Flitcraft A 1991 Spouse abuse. In: Rosenberg M, Fenley M A (eds) Violence in America. A public health approach. Oxford University Press, New York

Tayside Women and Violence Working Group 1994 Hit or miss. An exploratory study of the provision for women subjected to domestic violence in Tayside Region. Tayside Regional Council, Tayside

Turner B S 1995 Medical power and social knowledge, 2nd edn. Sage, London

Walker L E 1979 The battered woman. Harper and Row, New York

WHO 1946 Constitution. World Health Organisation, Geneva

Winstead-Fry P 1980 The scientific method and its impact on holistic health. Advanced Nursing Science 2: 1–7

Worcester N, Whatley M H 1992 The selling of HRT: playing on the fear factor. Feminist Review 41: 1–25

Zero Tolerance Trust 1992 Zero tolerance campaign. Zero Tolerance Trust, Edinburgh

6

Health for the population

Grace Lindsay

INTRODUCTION

In this chapter the concepts of health, disease and illness are reviewed for the purpose of highlighting the theoretical links with current health education and health promotion strategies. The focus of the chapter is population-based health, with the dimensions of health promotion approaches that have underpinned successful initiatives outlined. The World Health Organisation has provided a lead role in setting the Health for All targets together with the operationalisation of multidimensional, multiagency health promotion initiatives at an international level. Key messages from the Healthy Cities Projects are discussed in order to highlight the far-reaching approaches utilised as part of the implementation process in population-based health promotion.

The chapter concludes with a vision of the way forward to improve the health of the population. Health boards, in collaboration with key health-care practitioners, are leading the implementation of health improvement programmes to provide effective and efficiently delivered health care and a summary of their key objectives is presented.

HISTORICAL PERSPECTIVE

Hippocrates has been cited as the first individual to seek to explain the origins of disease, with many observations that remain relevant to health care today. He distinguished between diseases which were endemic (always present in a given area) and those which at times became excessively common (epidemic). He went further to suggest a role for exercise, diet, climate, water and the seasons as factors related to the development of disease and illness and as such was one of the first to highlight the interrelationship between humans and the environment.

From this early multifactorial view of determinants of health, a narrower perspective became popular in the 'germ' theory. The concept of disease embodied in the germ theory was the existence of a one-to-one relationship between the causal agent and disease. However, it was soon realised that a more complicated relationship existed for most diseases because, for example, although it was necessary to be exposed to the tubercular bacillus (TB) in order to develop pulmonary TB, not everyone who was exposed became infected. Thus, the realisation that some people developed a disease because of their nutritional status or their genetic make-up led to a 'seed and ground' model of causation which postulated an interplay between the causal agent and host. According to this theory, diseases could only flourish within an environment of adversity. This theory was quickly superseded by the modern view of cause, which is multifactorial.

Current understanding of the origins of disease has acknowledged that disease is rarely caused by a single agent alone but rather depends on a number of factors which combine to either produce the disease and illness or promote ill health. These factors can be grouped under the three headings of agent, host and environment and as such have provided the perspectives that underpin current approaches to the promotion of the health of the population.

HEALTH

Extensive debates have taken place and a great deal has been written about the concept of health and how it should be defined. It has been linked to the individual's social and cultural position which is shaped by experience, knowledge, values and expectations (Ewles & Simnett 1999). Perceptions of health have been shown to change over the course of life although there are some common elements. These include the ability to function, energy and vitality, psychosocial well-being and the understanding and recognition that high levels of health can be present despite a major illness (Blaxter 1990).

The World Health Organisation defines health as 'not merely the absence of disease and infirmity but complete physical, mental and social well-being' (WHO 1985). This definition was widely endorsed but is now relatively dated and has been criticised for several reasons. It described 'health' as a 'state' which implied that it was a fixed and static entity and was viewed as a Utopian ideal with few direct applications to individuals or populations in practice. However, it was considered an advance at that time because it introduced a multidimensional view of health and moved away from the absence of disease model. One of its important concepts was related to the possibility of high levels of health despite the presence of disease. More recently, the WHO has explored a variety of newer definitions of health, including 'a resource for living'.

The world of everyday life can therefore be viewed as the total sphere of an individual's experiences, being circumscribed by the objects of living and encompassing what is seen to be true or real to each individual. A clear understanding of the concept of health has been further complicated by terminology used to describe states of health and factors critical in determining health. These include the terms health, illness, disease and well-being, each presenting different perspectives.

ILL HEALTH AND DISEASE

The 'disease-based' view of ill health was founded on the premise that poor health was a function of an abnormality, with the term 'disease' used in a limited and scientific manner (Field 1976). Conversely, 'illness' was commonly used to describe a person's subjective experience of 'ill health' or 'disease' indicated by reported symptoms and subjective accounts, such as pain, distress or discomfort. Furthermore, objectively defined 'disease' does not bear a simple causal relationship with subjectively reported experience of illness. As MacIntyre (1986) noted, screening studies of random cross-sections of the population have shown that very few people are without some abnormalities that can be defined as 'disease', even though many of the affected individuals are unaware of the disorders. In a similar manner to the perspective of illness and disease, the term 'well-being' can also be viewed as a subjective view of the 'disease-free' health state.

In a qualitative study, the experience of feeling healthy for people living with a chronic illness and/or disability was explored in a group of eight individuals using an interpretive phenomenological approach. The essential attributes of feeling healthy identified by the participants were: honouring the self; seeking and connecting with others; creating opportunities; celebrating life; transcending the self; and acquiring a state of grace (Lindsey 1996). These positive experiences were not documented by previous work that examined the impact of chronic illness. Factors such as the sense of the loss of self-identity and strained and problematic relationships with others have been reported in work examining the influence of chronic disease to health (Charmaz 1997). A process of adaptation in order to cope has been identified and described as similar to that of grief (Matson 1977). In attempting to interpret the meaning of these differing perspectives of health within illness, it is important to consider also the focus of the research question. The different accounts that were given could be explained by simply changing the emphasis of the area of enquiry from that of 'health' to that of 'illness'.

In the Oxford Health Lifestyle Survey (Wright et al 1992) of those reporting long-term chronic illness, only 28% reported that their health was fair or poor on a scale of excellent, good, fair and poor. This highlights the complexities of assessing health where individuals are very well aware of the diseased state and yet rate their overall health as good which would suggest that people attach a complex meaning to this term 'health'. Many studies support the view that health should be regarded as a multi-dimensional concept that is not only the absence of disease, but a positive state of well-being and a reserve of overall health determined in large part by individual constitution (Herzlich 1973, Pill & Stott 1982, Blaxter 1985). Although health is generally characterised as a positive entity, individuals also have the ability to define health as coexisting with serious or long-term illness (Blaxter 1990). The paradox is clear in that individuals are perfectly capable of admitting to serious illness and yet claiming to be healthy and, on the other hand, there are those who report symptoms who have no discoverable pathology. There is a growing consensus that individuals have important knowledge of their own health state (Tuckett et al 1985) and therefore this view of health should be carefully recorded and monitored. This, in turn, has fuelled the search for better subjective measures of health.

HEALTH FROM A LAY PERSPECTIVE

Medical knowledge has been build upon the concept of disease whereas the lay perspective of health has been described as being rooted in the experience of illness, either personally or through others (Williams & Wood 1986). Lay beliefs about illness are many and varied and do not simply mirror medical science. Although this may imply that they lack any scientific and valid basis, they have been shown to be logical, consistent and coherent, providing narrative reconstructions of the relationship between illness and health (Williams & Popay 1996). Lay perspectives have been shown to bring together different aspects of people's experience of the onset, course and effects of their illness in an attempt to make sense of this in causal terms (Blaxter 1983). While the biological basis may be considered to shape and set limits on human experience, the recognition that 'it may tell us little about the social meaning and significance ascribed to such categories' has been cited as its major limitation in terms of understanding health (MacIntyre 1986).

DISEASE PREVENTION

Traditionally prevention has been classified into three types.

- Primary prevention, which seeks to actually prevent the onset of a disease.

- Secondary prevention, where the level of prevention aims to halt the progression of a disease once it is established. The critical issues here are early detection and early diagnosis, followed by prompt and effective treatment.
- Tertiary prevention is concerned with rehabilitation of people with an established disease to minimise residual disabilities and complication. Action taken at this stage aims at improving quality of life, even if the disease itself cannot be cured.

A preventive component of population-based health promotion programmes can involve specific interventions to reduce the risk of disease recurrence. Immunisation and vaccination programmes are an example of this primary prevention approach. In practice, specific preventive techniques will often be used in combination with another element of health promotion. In this example, health education would be an essential component in order to raise parents' awareness of the benefits of immunisation and encourage them to bring their children into the programme.

HEALTH PROMOTION OR EDUCATION?

The terms 'health promotion' and 'health education' have been used in some cases to mean the same entity whereas in other cases they have been viewed as ideologically different. However, a degree of consensus has emerged within the published literature (Benson & Latter 1998), with health education being viewed as focusing on the individual lifestyle and health promotion focusing on structural, fiscal and ecological dimensions. It is acknowledged that both elements should be present in a comprehensive health promotion strategy (Macdonald & Bunton 1992).

The traditional approach to health education has been described as authoritarian, prescriptive and persuasive with dissemination of information from the 'expert' to the 'ignorant' (Tones & Telford 1994). In contrast, the 'new paradigm' of health promotion is based on a client-centred approach that is collaborative and utilises empowerment as a central concept in motivation to improve health-related activities. The latter approach has been described as 'ethically more justifiable' (French & Adams 1986), having a sound theoretical basis (Tones 1987) and the generation of a growing body of empirical evidence to demonstrate its effectiveness (Beattie 1991).

HEALTH PROMOTION
Ideology

The modern public health movement began to take shape in the early 1970s and was based upon the ideals of improving health and tackling some of the seemingly intractable problems of chronic disease and its consequences.

The publication of the Health of the Nation White Paper in the early 1990s (DoH 1992) raised the profile of health improvement as a national priority. It firmly established that the health of the population as well as the care of patients should be specifically addressed.

In the context of health promotion, health has been considered 'less as an abstract state and more in terms of the ability to achieve one's potential and to respond positively to the challenges of the environment' (De Leeuw 1989). Health promotion has been described as:

- the process of fostering awareness, influencing attitudes and identifying alternatives so that individuals can make informed choices and change their behaviour to achieve an optimum level of physical and mental health, and improve their physical and social environment (CINHAL 1992);
- the process of enabling people to increase control over the determinants of health and thereby improve their health (WHO 1985);
- the organised application of educational, social and environmental resources enabling individuals to adopt and maintain behaviours that reduce risk of disease and enhance wellness (Petosa 1986).

Some common ground exists within these definitions, generating a consensus that health promotion may be regarded as a process that encompasses disease management, disease prevention, health education and the politics of health. However, it should be remembered that just as health itself means different things to different people, the concept of health promotion may equally be interpreted widely with different emphases placed on its individual components. In practice, the term 'health promotion', used alone or in combination with disease prevention, embraces a wide variety of perspectives from preventing premature death to legislative and physical measures to improve health, the promotion of individuals' responsibility for the maintenance of healthy ways of living and mobilising the support of communities as part of health improvement programmes. Reducing the risk of disease, premature death or illness and disability or any other undesirable health event is the orientation of preventive activity within the health promotion process.

Empowerment

The concept of empowerment is central to the philosophy and practice of health promotion. In one sense, it parallels the concept of health in that it can be said to be both a desirable end in itself and a means to an end. Empowerment of individuals and communities acts instrumentally to facilitate healthy decision making. It has to do with the relationship between individuals and their environment where the relationship is recognised to be reciprocal. At the micro level empowerment is also a key health promotion goal. For instance, as part of planned contract behaviour modification, people might learn how to avoid environmental circumstances which trigger their consumption of tobacco or alcohol. They might acquire skills in resisting social pressure and provide clear examples how the rhetoric of empowerment can be operationalised and translated into specific educational objectives. Self-empowerment concepts include beliefs about control, e.g. perceived locus of control and self-efficacy beliefs, values such as self-esteem and a variety of specific social and personal skills which might be encapsulated in the term 'health and life skills' (Sidell & Peberdy 1987, p. 40).

Health promotion in practice

In the last 20 years there have been major developments in preventive medicine, fuelled by an increasing acceptance in medical and political circles that the common chronic diseases of middle and later life constitute the principal health issues of industrialised societies. This movement has become characterised by the emergence of a clear policy agenda based on the management of mass behaviour change. These developments have brought to the fore the concept of lifestyle, a loose aggregation of behaviours and conditions encompassing body size, shape, diet, exercise and the use of drugs, both legal and illegal. Improving the lifestyle of the population soon became the major challenge deemed necessary to improve the health of the population and was first entrusted to a professional grouping initially known as 'health education' and later as 'health promotion'. The movement to change the lifestyle of the population attracted severe criticism because if a disease is preventable by adopting or avoiding certain behaviours, then it follows that victims of such disorders are at least partially to blame for their predicament. A recurring theme in the critiques of behavioural preventive medicine questions the processes and evidence that attribute a specific proportion of disease to lifestyle causes (Davey Smith & Shipley 1991).

Incorporation of lifestyle factors into systems for delivering health thus comprises a change in the ways that population groups encounter health care and indeed in the forms that providing for health takes. Health promotion programmes are designed to persuade individuals to purchase or adopt different types of lifestyle, depending upon their degree of consumer power, including both their financial capacity to acquire particular goods and services and also their status as champion or potentially powerful exemplar of a particular lifestyle. The term 'lifestyle' has recently come to be used widely in many contexts. Apart from its direct association with health-related behaviour, it has been used to denote general conditions of living, as a product brand name and to describe a type of television programme.

One of the major problems facing the professions and institutions involved at the behavioural end of contemporary preventive medicine is the apparent failure of many individuals to comply fully with healthy lifestyle advice. In the developing discourse of health education, this situation has been attributed to two major causes. In the first place, it was suggested that there was a lack of accurate knowledge among the general public concerning the potential harm associated with certain aspects of everyday behaviour (Health Education News 1981), so that people who had heart disease could be seen as victims of their own ignorance. This perspective assumed that if knowledge were increased, rational people would decide to change their daily habits. A second more sophisticated line of analysis suggests that the major cause of non-compliance is the existence of an attitude which sees health as being largely determined by forces outside the control of the individual and thus denies the possible relevance of personal behavioural change. This approach has led to the idea that health promotion has been involved in a battle for the 'hearts and minds' of the population, a struggle between a modern belief in lifestyle and a culture of fatalism (Pill & Stott 1987).

Society's health is not just an individual responsibility. Health, to a large extent, has been governed by the physical, social, cultural and economic environment in which we live and work. To focus exclusively on changing individual behaviours to the exclusion of environmental circumstances has been described as a fundamentally defective strategy (Tones & Telford 1994). For these reasons the process of building a healthy public policy is at the very heart of health promotion. Because traditional preventive models of health education place great emphasis on individual lifestyle changes, this may encourage 'victim blaming' since it has often been the case that social and environmental factors create unhealthy circumstances in the first place.

A more radical approach has been envisaged that seeks to bring about social and political change in order to make the healthy choices a more viable option. The radical option is fully compatible with the Ottawa Charter which brought the matter of health policy centre stage and argued that there would be a global improvement in health only when governments made serious attempts to deal with environmental and social circumstances which militated against health and nurtured disease.

IMPROVING THE HEALTH OF THE POPULATION

A landmark international WHO conference on health promotion held in Ottawa in 1986 considered lifestyles conducive to health and the consensus generated was published as the Ottawa Charter for Health Promotion (WHO 1986). The Charter has outlined a comprehensive strategy for health promotion with five dimensions.

- Healthy public policy
- Supportive environments
- Personal skills

- Community action
- Reoriented health services

The Charter was an important influence on the value and emphasis placed on the term 'health' and its determinants. The Charter's objectives reached beyond the domain of the traditional health services with broader terms of reference and much more emphasis placed on health, as opposed to illness. The WHO perspective can be summarised as follows.

Health is a holistic entity, a positive state which is essential for individuals to achieve a socially and economically productive life. Health gain will be achieved and illness prevented through the eradication of health inequalities between and within nations and social groups.

Programmes to improve health have become much more wide ranging and have placed greater emphasis on individuals' perception of their own health status but have stressed the importance of psychological, social and environmental measures in achieving true health improvement in populations. This broader view of promoting health, while acknowledging the importance of improving lifestyles, health services and environment, recognises that more fundamental conditions need to be met if high levels of health in populations are to be attained. A healthy nation is one which has an equitable distribution of resources but also one which has active empowered communities involved in creating conditions necessary for a healthy people.

However, health is not just an individual's responsibility: our health, to a large extent, is governed by the physical, social, cultural and economic environments in which we live and work. The building of healthy public policy is at the very heart of health promotion (Tones & Telford 1994, pp. 4–5). A reorientation of the health services has started to take place to reflect the wide range of public, voluntary and private services that have an important role in the promotion of health through enabling, not coercing, and a focus clearly on cooperation rather than compliance. Against this broad background, the 'new public health' can therefore be summarised as a panoptic term for those individuals, movements, ideas and strategies that seek to decrease absolute and relative social inequalities in health through a concurrent emphasis upon the modification of personal behaviour, the amelioration of adverse environmental factors and the more equitable provision of resources related to health.

Another WHO strategy is that of Health for All (WHO 1985) which was based on the principle of equity. The first 12 items set specific quantifiable targets in terms of improvements in health status sought over the 20-year period from 1980 to 2000 based on the Health for All strategy. They can be grouped into three categories: the basic Health for All goals, the health of vulnerable populations and specific health problems. The health outcomes within these targets have four interrelated themes.

- *Ensuring equity in health* – through reduction in health status differences between countries and between groups within countries.
- *Adding life to years* – helping people to achieve, and use, their full physical, mental and social potential.
- *Adding health to life* – through reducing disease and disability and providing good health care accessible to all.
- *Adding years to life* – through increasing life expectancy.

The strategies outlined in order to meet these objectives address changes in lifestyles, improvements in the environment and developments in prevention, treatment and care that will make their achievement possible. National, regional and local initiatives were proposed whose objectives were to actively support healthy living patterns such as balanced nutrition and appropriate physical activity and reductions in consumption of excess alcohol, cigarette smoking and drugs. In addition to acknowledging the importance of improving people's knowledge of and motivation for health through health education, the Health for All policy gives major emphasis to changes in social, economic, cultural, physical and other factors that influence the health-related choices made by individuals, groups and communities. The targets promoted by the WHO present challenges for politicians and those in positions of power to achieve reductions in social differences in health while promoting equal health opportunities for all (Touros 1989).

HEALTHY CITIES PROJECT
Background

The WHO Healthy Cities Project (WHO 1990) is an example of social policy designed to address the disparities in health status between different social groups. The principle that all people have an equal right to health is the foundation of the project. The activities promoted by this initiative focus on altering the social and physical environment, providing the means to support healthy lifestyles and ensuring services are available to all.

Changing the physical and social environment requires broad policies aimed at structural developments in working and living environments. Policies to enable healthy lifestyles centre on reducing lifestyle risks through health education combined with treating the fundamental conditions affecting lifestyle. Action to ensure that services are accessible to all concentrate on eliminating barriers to services, whether they be cultural, organisational, financial or environmental. The role of local government is central to the Healthy Cities concept and one that distinguishes it from other community-level health promotion programmes. There are over 1000 Healthy Cities projects established throughout the world, including every WHO region.

Assessment of need across these cities identified common problems such as ageing, migrants, cardiovascular disease and cancer, economic decline, inadequate housing and traffic. Operational characteristics included community assessment, communication and information exchange and training of various categories of workers to promote health. Development of city health plans and technical and financial assistance were provided to community groups to start action throughout the city or in specific neighbourhood localities. Promotion of public health policy has been noted as central to the Healthy Cities approach.

In practice

Four common approaches have been adopted in terms of addressing policy change. These include: adoption of position statements to advocate for city council resolutions; facilitation of the adoption of policies on particular health issues; targeting of specific population groups, geographic areas or services formulation and adoption of comprehensive city health plans. Finally, they advocate for assessments of the impact of city policies on health and the use of assessments by decision makers. Characteristics of successful Healthy Cities projects have been identified as – effective leadership; multisectorial Healthy Cities steering groups to direct the projects; a strong economy; community participation; information used in city-wide planning; obtaining appropriate technical support; being viewed as a credible resource for health in the community; effective networking; smaller city size or neighbourhoods in large cities. The majority of projects are located within city administration departments and not in designated health centres or hospitals.

No consensus exists on the best indicators of success of the Healthy Cities Project despite considerable effort to construct a valid set. Reasons for the uncertainty have been given as the lack of relevance of indicators to health promotion; use of static methods of attempting to measure dynamic community processes; questionable validity of applying indicators to compare cities that have different physical, social, political and cultural contexts; and different local needs and priorities. The project has generated a plethora of official and 'unofficial' schemes. The latter are intended to implement Health for All principles at the level of cities, towns and even villages and to develop new models of 'good' practice. These projects have differed markedly although the operational approach has been largely at the level of local government, municipal health and environmental agencies with involvement of local voluntary and community groups (WHO Regional Office for Europe 1990). Projects under the Healthy Cities banner appear, initially, to diverge considerably in terms of scope, objectives and intended outcomes. The Drumchapel Healthy Cities Project, for example, has concentrated on facilitating or building upon individual community health actions such as a forum for clients with mental health problems and an intersectoral 'HIV and addictions' group. This example of community development illustrated the implementation of policy into practice provided by a community development project conducted in an area of high socioeconomic deprivation near Glasgow (Craig 1996). The process commenced with a community health profile to identify key health issues with community residents. The profile groups included local residents and fieldworkers from various agencies and projects. The main findings from the community profile were that environmental and housing issues were priority areas. Key health issues identified were: cold and damp housing; traffic and lack of play areas for children; high rates of cigarette smoking with half of the smokers indicating that they would like to stop; emotional difficulties or difficulty sleeping. The project provided support and training for local people to work as 'community health volunteers' to help address these identified local health needs. These roles involved participation in or facilitating community health activities such as local health needs assessment, health forums and self-help groups together with raising awareness of health issues and helping to shape the agenda and direction of the project. The other aims of the project were to develop mechanisms for community participation and collaborative working on local health issues, to extend the scope of community health activity by supporting new and existing community health forums.

Evaluation and dissemination of the activities of the project were undertaken. Self-help groups have been established for asthma sufferers, postnatal women and bereavement counselling. Community health forums facilitated by the project include a women's health network, a food action group, a community drugs forum and a new health forum to develop a health strategy for the area.

Other cities have sought to coordinate their responses to particular problems, e.g. Patras, Griefswald and Horsens decided in 1992 to research noise pollution with the aim of revising policies in such areas as traffic routing and selective traffic curfews. Beyond the official Healthy Cities, there have been programmes of multisectoral action in the fields of health promotion, community consultation and movement towards an integrated 'healthy public policy', most notable within the UK in Sheffield.

HEALTH PROMOTION DISSEMINATION

The use of mass media approaches for the promotion of health has assisted both social advocacy, such as promoting organisational and environmental change, and personal education, such as facilitating individual and group behaviour change. These are often disseminated through large-scale campaigns to populations of several millions utilising paid advertising, commissioned programmes and news items. The outlets vary and comprise television, radio and newspapers together with posters, leaflets and books. Increasingly, multimedia information systems including the WorldWide Web are used by large groups of the population as a means of communi-

---

Box 6.1   Population strategies for health promotion dissemination

- Increasing general public and political awareness
- Providing healthy living information and advice
- Presentation of a corporate image
- Changing attitudes by presenting examples and role models
- Introducing skills and encouraging self-confidence
- Offering triggers and incentives for action and participation
- Promotion of specific activities, events or opportunities
- Encouraging maintenance of behaviour change
- Broadcasting achievements and successes to reward action

---

cation and entertainment and as a source of information. This is particularly true for the younger age groups.

The key objectives contained within population-focused health promotion dissemination are summarised in Box 6.1.

EVALUATION OF HEALTH PROMOTION

Defining boundaries for health promotion activities has been difficult and it has been suggested that for practical purposes it may be considered as 'an approach to any interaction or activity which is characterised by certain key features' (Cribb & Dines 1993). The key features referred to, summarised in Box 6.2, are a useful starting point for thinking about how health promotion activities will be evaluated.

Little research has been conducted on the wide range of factors that may impinge on outcome determination within the context of health promotional interventions. The answers to three broad questions are helpful in guiding identification of suitable endpoints for evaluation.

What should be measured?

The goals of the specific intervention must be identified and made explicit. These are likely to include both process, such as attendance rates at classes, and outcome measures, such as smoking cessation rates.

Box 6.2   Key activities in health promotion

• Holism	• Individualisation
• Equity	• Negotiation
• Participation	• Facilitation
• Collaboration	• Support

How will outcomes be determined and measured?

These will vary according to the client's and nurse's perspectives. The majority of clients are attempting to alter their lifestyle in a positive manner through behaviour change. This is unlikely to happen in one single step but rather as a series of intermediate steps from increased awareness of the need to change to increased motivation to make changes followed by a series of change attempts and finally success in altering lifestyle practices. This cyclical process has been described by Prochaska & Diclemente (1984) and suggests that clients will be at different stages of change at any given time and therefore different nursing interventions will be appropriate at various times. This implies that blanket approaches to health promotion through mass media campaigns are likely to have limited impact because of the different needs of individuals at the various stages of behavioural change.

When is the appropriate time to measure outcomes?

The timing of data collection is often critical to the results. Data collected too soon after the intervention may not accurately reflect the outcome state or capture the subtle changes in the client's understanding, attitude, perceptions and motivation to undertake change. In addition, possible explanatory variables relating to the process of the intervention that are helpful in identification of possible reasons for success or failure are also omitted. However, data collected too long after the intervention make it difficult to isolate the main effect of the intervention as opposed to other confounding variables. Multiple measures of outcome at various time periods before and after interventions are therefore advocated. A summary of stages of outcome assessment, highlighting suitable parameters that would be useful as indicators of change, is presented in Box 6.3.

Although the types and timing of the outcome assessment can be guided by the general categories of outcomes outlined in Box 6.3, in practice several

---

Box 6.3 Stages and variables in health promotion outcome assessment (adapted from Gillis 1995)

Immediate outcomes	*Intermediate outcomes*	*Final outcomes*
Reduced risk factors	Maintenance of healthy	Reduced illness
Enhanced well-being,	lifestyle behaviour	Extended longevity
e.g. stamina, energy,	Improved performance	Improved quality of life
concentration	Improved fitness and	Lowered mortality rates
Effective coping	self-confidence	
Organisational and	Improved self-esteem and	
environmental change	self-efficiency	
	Reduced medical utilisation	

difficulties become apparent. In particular, some of the concepts are not readily measurable, such as self-esteem or self-confidence, and others such as extended longevity would require large numbers of individuals and a considerable study time before a meaningful evaluation could be undertaken. In this latter example, extended longevity is often implied by the impact of improved lifestyle behaviour, such as smoking cessation. Health outcome measurement has been addressed in more detail in Chapter 12.

NURSING EDUCATION AND HEALTH

Nursing can best fulfil its potential in primary health care when nursing education provides a sound foundation for nursing practice, especially work in the community, and when nurses take account of the social aspects of health needs and have a broader understanding of health development (European Conference on Nursing 1989). In partnership with the WHO, the Association of Schools of Public Health in the European Region is producing curricula and learning materials for use in public health training based on Health for All. The aim is to develop postgraduate vocational studies in a multidisciplinary field which encompass disease prevention, health protection and promotion programmes for populations and for the organisation of high-quality cost-effective health services, with a particular stress on leadership, policy making, management and communication skills. It has been suggested that these topics be taught within an integrated curriculum because, for example, communication skills in themselves have no inherent value. An open question, for instance, is neither 'good' or 'bad'; its value is entirely dependent upon the context in which the case of the nurse/patient interaction is linked to therapeutic intent (Benson & Latter 1998).

It has been suggested that the extent to which nurses experience empowerment themselves may be a crucial determinant of the extent to which they are able to foster this in patients (Benson & Latter 1998). This explanation has been supported by work examining student nurses' attitudes and experience of health promotion in practice. The results highlighted the following key areas that identify barriers to health promotion activities in practice.

- Students report a lack of role models in practice.
- A view from practitioners and patients that health promotion is only an issue for healthy people.
- The need for nurses themselves to be empowered in order to empower others.
- Within nurse education, there was a lack of integration of interpersonal skills with health promotion thereby failing to reinforce the value of such skills as part of the promotion of health.

Health promotion at a population level is a multiagency, multidisciplinary activity and for nursing to contribute in this arena, the barriers to practice highlighted in Benson & Latter (1998) need to be addressed

THE FUTURE

The National Health Service, through its structure of health boards, NHS trusts, primary care practitioners and other workers, aims to provide efficient and effective care for patients. In order to achieve these goals health boards, trusts, clinicians and general practitioners are working together to produce health improvement programmes for the population of each health board area. Each health improvement plan should cover a 5-year period and include proposals to:

- protect the public health, including emergency planning;
- promote the health of its population;
- analyse and tackle health inequalities;
- provide a rolling programme for the implementation and monitoring of evidence-based clinical guidelines and clinically effective practice;
- employ human resources and existing assets efficiently;
- integrate information management and technology systems to improve communication and utilisation of important health data.

Health improvement programmes will address clinical priorities which will be reviewed and updated as necessary. At present, these priorities are mental health, coronary heart disease and stroke and cancer. The health improvement programmes approach has stressed the importance of the need to focus on health gain and improved outcomes for local populations.

CONCLUSION

Health promotion in practice is an organised, multidimensional, multiagency activity. It involves many strategies including health education, health maintenance and protection, community and environmental development, research and healthy public policy. Health promotion can be viewed as a means to an end: a distinct entity in health care to achieve the targets outlined within the WHO Health for All recommendations. In practical terms, improving the health of local populations will be undertaken in a collaborative manner as part of the broader remit of health improvement programmes which will be led by health boards with the focus on the population of that area.

REFERENCES

Beattie A 1991 Knowledge and control in health promotion: a test case for social policy and social theory. In: Gabe J, Calnan M, Bury M (eds) The sociology of the health service. Routledge, London

Benson A, Latter S 1998 Implementing health promoting nursing: the integration of interpersonal skills and health promotion. Journal of Advanced Nursing 27: 100–107

Blaxter M 1983 The causes of disease. Women talking. Social Science and Medicine 17(2): 59–69

Blaxter M 1985 Self definition of health status and consulting rates in primary care. Quarterly Journal of Social Affairs 1: 131–171

Blaxter M 1990 Health and lifestyles. Routledge, London

Charmaz K 1997 Loss of self: a fundamental form of suffering in the chronically ill. Sociology of Health and Illness 5(2): 168–198

CINHAL 1992 CINHAL Information Systems, Glendale, CA

Craig P 1996 Drumming up health in Drumchapel: community development health visiting. Health Visitor 69(11): 459–461

Cribb A, Dines A 1993 What is health promotion? In: Dines A, Cribb A (eds) Health promotion: concepts and practice. Blackwell Science, Oxford

Davey Smith G, Shipley M 1991 Confounding of occupation and smoking: its magnitude and consequences. Social Science and Medicine 32: 1297–1300

Department of Health (DoH) 1992 The health of the nation. HMSO, London

De Leeuw E 1989 Concepts in health promotion: the notion of relativism. Social Science and Medicine 29: 1281–1288

European Conference on Nursing 1989 Report on a WHO meeting. WHO regional Office for Europe, Copenhagen

Ewles L, Simnett I 1999 Promoting health: a practical guide, 4th edn. Baillière Tindall, London

Field D 1976 The social definition of illness. In: Tuckett D (ed) An introduction to medical sociology. Tavistock, London, pp 334–365

French J, Adams L 1986 From analysis to synthesis: theories of health education. Health Education Journal 45(2): 71–74

Gillis A 1995 Exploring nursing outcomes for health promotion. Nursing Forum 30(2): 5–12

Health Education News 1981 Heart disease risks ignored. Health Education Council, London

Herzlich C 1973 Health and illness. Academic Press, London

Lindsay E 1996 Health within illness: experiences of chronically ill/disabled. Journal of Advanced Nursing 24: 465–472

Macdonald G, Bunton R 1992 Health promotion: discipline or disciples? In: Bunton R, Macdonald G (eds) Health promotion: disciplines and diversity. Routledge, London

MacIntyre S 1986. Health and illness. In: Burgess R G (ed) Key variables in social investigation. Routledge and Kegan Paul, London, pp 99–122

Matson R R 1977 Adjustment to multiple sclerosis: an exploratory study. Social Science and Medicine 11: 245–250

Petosa R 1986 Emerging trends in adolescent health promotion. Health Values 10(3): 22–28

Pill R, Stott N 1982 Concept of illness causation and responsibility: some preliminary data from a sample of working class mothers. Social Science and Medicine 16: 43–52

Pill R, Stott N 1987 Development of a measure of potential behaviour: a Salience and Lifestyle Index. Social Science and Medicine 24(2): 125–134

Prochaska J O, Diclemente C C 1984 The transtheoretical approach: crossing traditional foundations of change. Don Jones, Irwin, Homewood, IL

Sidell M, Peberdy A (eds) 1987 Debates and dilemmas in promoting health: a reader. Open University/Macmillan Press, Basingstoke

Tones K 1987 Promoting health: the contribution of education. Paper presented at the World Health Organisation Consultation on Co-ordinated Infrastructure for Health Education, Copenhagen

Tones B, Telford S (eds) 1994 Health education: effectiveness, efficiency and equity. Chapman and Hall, London, pp 4–5

Touros A D 1989 Equity and the Healthy Cities project. Health Promotion 4(2): 73–75

Tuckett D, Boulton M, Olson C, Williams A 1985 Meetings between experts. Tavistock, London

WHO 1985 Targets for health for all. WHO Regional Office for Europe, Copenhagen

WHO 1986 Ottowa Charter of Health Promotion. Geneva, WHO

WHO 1990 Healthy Cities Project: a project becomes a movement. WHO Regional Office for Europe, SOGESS, Milan

Williams G, Popay J 1996 Lay knowledge and the privilege of experience. In: Gabe J, Kelleher D, Williams G (eds) Challenging medicine. Routledge, London, pp 118–139

Williams G H, Wood P H N 1986 Common-sense beliefs about illness: a mediating role for the doctor. Lancet ii: 1435–1437

Wright L D, Harwood A, Coulter A 1992 Health and lifestyles in the Oxford Region. Health Services Research Unit, Oxford

Nursing elements of public health

SECTION CONTENTS

7

Nursing for the community: assessing and meeting individual and population health needs

Jean B McIntosh

INTRODUCTION

The process of assessing people's health needs has to operate at a number of different levels including the individual, the practice and the wider population. The assessment of health needs also takes place within the context of professional views about how needs assessment should be conducted, within a framework of policy guidelines and in a climate of resource constraint. It is also the case that if there is confusion about the public health nursing role, as detailed in Chapter 1, then assessment of need in the public health arena could be unclear.

Thus the development and use of effective systems of needs assessment are not straightforward. If community nurses' assessments of need are influenced significantly by resource constraints or by disagreements about the nature of need or the meaning of health, then it follows that there will be dissension about their role and also about the appropriate emphasis of their work. It is important therefore to explore the process of community nursing assessment of need in order to identify the ways in which this activity is shaped by nurses and others and what potential consequences this has for their contribution to the health of the population.

This chapter considers some of the difficulties associated with assessing need in order to highlight the theoretical and practical problems for community nursing interventions at the individual and population level. The chapter will begin with an exploration of the policy aspects of needs assessment and will go on to consider the concept of need and then explore more closely the implications of these issues for community nursing.

THE POLICY VIEW OF NEEDS ASSESSMENT

The problems associated with assessment of patient and client health need in the community differ according to whether the focus is on care during episodes of ill health or the maintenance or improvement of good health. In relation to a focus on ill health, the problems associated with needs assessment were brought into sharp focus by the introduction of the 1990 NHS and Community Care Act (DoH 1990). Prior to the Act, the Griffiths Report, *Community care – agenda for action*, had for the first time identified principles for the assessment process. These principles included the assessment of individuals in the context of their own situation, ensuring that patient/client wishes were taken into account and also involving the prioritisation of each case according to the resources available. These are the essential ingredients of a needs-led rather than a service-led approach to assessment (Griffiths 1988). They sprang from a belief that professional or normative constructions of need were substantially out of touch with patient- or client-defined need and this was true of both health and social care professionals (Smith 1980, Badger et al 1988, Luker & Perkins 1988).

These principles were subsequently endorsed by the White Paper *Caring for people* and eventually enshrined within the NHS and Community Care Act of 1990 which gave lead responsibility to Social Services and Social Work departments for assessment of need and its subsequent management (DHSS 1989). Detailed guidelines about assessment processes were outlined and these were to be separated from actual care delivery (DoH/SSI 1991). This policy view of needs assessment ushered in an important anomaly.

The twin requirements to take account of patient/client wishes and to prioritise according to resource constraints are incompatible unless patient/client wishes exactly coincide with the services available to them. The inevitable corollary of an assessment which encourages patients and clients to offer an unrestricted view of their needs and wishes is unfulfilled expectations and, in the social service field, the potential threat of legal action (Cervi 1993). The authors of the policy documents outlined above failed to anticipate such problems and, more importantly, ignored the professional processes already in place which manage assessment in such a way as to identify needs and also to negotiate which needs can be addressed. Such negotiation has led to the professional or normative view of need becoming the dominant force within assessment, as the research cited above has shown. However, it could be argued that if the process of negotiation could be developed in a more patient/client-centred manner, then the assessment process would be more open and sensitive without incurring the risk of uncovering needs which cannot be met. The issue, then, is not one of reconstituting the framework of assessment but rather trying to identify how assessment can embody best practice in terms of sensitive negotiation between practitioners and patient/client.

A different set of difficulties confronts practitioners in assessing health needs which relate to the achievement, maintenance or improvement of good health. First among these is the difficulty of definition and the fact that health may be interpreted differently by different groups. As Robinson (1985) has argued, the diffuseness of the concept of health and the problems associated with its measurement make it an uncertain basis for professional activity. This problem has also been highlighted by Cowley (1995, p. 435) whose grounded theory study offered evidence that health is viewed by health visitors as a process which involves individuals accumulating and using 'resources for health'. As Cowley points out, this view does not sit comfortably with the need to respond to setting and achieving measurable health promotion targets.

Second, there is the tension between the medical and social models of health, whereby the broad thrust of medically dominated initiatives emphasises the identification of disease risk factors and the means by which these may be reduced, while the social model of health focuses on factors such as poverty and deprivation as powerful determinants of health (see Chapter 5).

As a consequence of definition problems and the tension between different models of health, it is not surprising that addressing health promotion needs and public health needs poses a number of difficulties for practitioners.

First, the degree of emphasis which should be placed on working at the level of the individual and the level of effort which should be directed at the community or population are not clear. Moreover, as Craig points out in Chapter 1, the structural conditions for developing a public health contribution have been slow to develop. However the publication of the White Papers *Saving lives: our healthier nation* (for England and Wales) and *Towards a healthier Scotland* may lessen some of these difficulties (DoH 1999, SODoH 1999). Both White Papers contain an explicit focus on the social causes of disease and ill health and adopt a broad cross-sectoral approach to the improvements in public health. Importantly, they also identify the potential for health visitors to have a better defined public health role.

The ability to assess health need at the level of the community and the population is therefore of paramount importance given these new policy initiatives. However, as needs assessment is not a straightforward process, it is important to explore the concept of need in order to see how it might be interpreted by community nurses in their assessment practice.

UNDERSTANDING THE CONCEPT OF NEED

The term 'need' is problematic as it has widely varying interpretations. For example, some authors use the term to describe deficits in functioning while others define it as the ability to benefit from a service; it has also been argued that need statements are social constructs which depend on the perspectives and values of those who make them (Bradshaw 1972, Doyal & Gough 1991, Seedhouse 1994).

The philosopher Liss has analysed the meaning of health care need in some detail, identifying the structure of need in terms of a state (the health problem), a goal (resolving the health problem) and the means of moving from the state to the goal (the specific intervention to resolve the problem) (Liss 1993). In public health terms, the same framework could be applied but in this case the state might be the absence of a healthy lifestyle among groups within a population and the goal the achievement of a healthy or healthier lifestyle. Liss argues that information about the state, the goal and the means of reaching the goal is a necessary and sufficient requirement for a need assessment to take place.

This approach is echoed in part in the work of McWalter who argues that needs assessment is not simply a compilation of a set of problems or difficulties. Rather, it is a two-stage process involving not only the identification of health problems but also the determining of the nature of care, support or action required to resolve or alleviate those problems (McWalter et al 1994). In other words, there is a recognition of the state and the means of reaching the goal to address the problem although the goal itself is left implicit.

The fact that needs assessment is not necessarily a straightforward process is acknowledged by Liss when he notes that while the state can be regarded as 'factual' and capable of being described by empirical observation, the goal is chosen and thus subject to different views held by those involved, namely patients/clients, carers and professionals. Furthermore, the means of reaching the goal may also involve value-laden decisions. Thus the process of negotiation and the reconciling of different views, as referred to above, clearly constitutes an important element in the needs assessment process.

In exploring the utility to community nursing of this model of needs assessment, it is important to consider how it fits with the varying areas of responsibility of the different specialist groups. Thus it is important to ask whether the notions of verifiable state, selected goals and means of achieving those goals illuminate the current needs assessment challenges confronting community nurses. In particular, how far can public health issues such as primary and secondary prevention be understood in terms of verifiable states? Are goals always consciously chosen and how much freedom do practitioners have in selecting the means to achieve their goals?

ASSESSING PUBLIC HEALTH NEEDS

Health visiting

The health visitor's role incorporates primary, secondary and tertiary prevention. In relation to the scope of the interventions included in these three areas of preventive work, how far is it possible for health visitors to define the group or groups which would benefit from their intervention? What strategies do they use to identify the verifiable states which merit the setting of goals and subsequent health-visiting action?

As Chalmers states, there is no empirical evidence which identifies the methods used by health visitors to conceptualise needs or the practice strategies used to search out needs (Chalmers 1993). In her research, Chalmers found that although different processes were used to elicit information from clients, practitioners appeared to operate according to their own frameworks for practice which in turn guided how they allocated time and resources. Given the fact that health visitors work with individuals, families and community groups in a wide range of different settings, this variation of approach is not surprising.

Other research also suggests that the process of identifying need and allocating resources by health visitors does not appear to have a rational basis. For example, Shepherd (1992) examined health-visiting caseloads in Bristol by using a 26-factor checklist which emphasised 'social' needs and found that health visitors with greater needs on their caseloads were not compensated with smaller caseloads. A similar project is described by Powell in which clients' needs were rated according to physical, emotional and socioeconomic factors and caseloads and workloads were analysed to identify any anomalies in order to ensure that those clients with greater scores were given more health-visiting time (Powell 1995).

While the lack of a needs assessment framework appears to lead to certain anomalies, efforts made by management to refocus health-visiting activity can be similarly lacking a rational basis. In one major Scottish city, the introduction of a health-visiting protocol which advised a limit of five visits to the preschool child was an attempt to reduce the alleged level of unnecessary intervention with this group, thereby freeing health visitors for other work. This was clearly a population-based approach to addressing need but it was introduced without consultation with practitioners and while it was seen to have some benefits, it also incurred a range of difficulties which have been described elsewhere (Carney et al 1996).

It is clear, then, that the systems which health visitors use to identify need at the individual level need to be evaluated. It is also the case that managers or others who seek to shift the focus of health-visiting intervention towards a client group with a different range of needs require a rationale for so doing. This is of key importance owing to the fact that health visitors have a dual role and are required to fulfil elements of their preventive work at the level of the population.

The dual role and the assessment of need

There has been a long-standing debate both within and outside the profession as to how best to fulfil the dual role of the health visitor involving work at the public health and the individual client levels (Fatchett 1990). The challenges involved in the assumption of this dual role are exemplified in Twinn's discussion of conflicting paradigms in health-visiting practice (Twinn 1991). If the mainstay of health-visiting work is at the individual level of the child, how do health visitors work at the level of the community or population and how is the need for such activity assessed?

Central to health-visiting education and policy is the use of the community profile, in which a social, economic and epidemiological profile of a practitioner's or group of practitioners' area is compiled (Luker & Orr 1992, Hawtin et al 1994). The Health Visitors' Association produces comprehensive guidelines on the compilation of such profiles and the literature suggests the need to target certain client groups (Twinn et al 1990). The use of the community profile has been questioned within the profession in relation to its methodological weaknesses and in particular, the value of 'hard' statistics as opposed to the 'softer' data such as practitioner knowledge of attitudes and lifestyles has been challenged (Cernik & Wearne 1992, Thomas 1997). Such qualitative data are often unwritten and unacknowledged but may add an important dimension to the understanding of a community's complex needs. However, the production of individual community profiles is time consuming and likely to result in a fragmented approach to this aspect of the health visitor's dual role.

The complexity of undertaking a proper community-based assessment of health needs has been identified by Schultz & Magilvy (1998) who used a combination of three strategies – research-based surveys, ethnographic methods and census data – to show that the three in combination provided the different levels of information necessary to develop a health programme for the community. Similar conclusions were drawn by Ong et al (1991) in their work on community-based rapid appraisal of community health needs and also by Murray & Graham (1995). There is a recognition that needs assessment should be undertaken within a social rather than a medical model of health promotion.

There is ample evidence that health visitors do in fact target certain groups and the plethora of initiatives aimed at improving the public's health is evident in reports of health-visiting activity (McIntosh et al 1994). An overview of health promotion activity at the level of the community was undertaken in Glasgow by Craig who found that two-thirds of the reported examples of health promotion activity focused on the health board-stated priorities for health (Craig 1995, unpublished paper). However, there is a wide variety of competing and conflicting claims upon the time of health visitors and some choice between them is necessary. How health visitors make such choices is not clear and it is a moot point whether they stem from community profiles, from practitioners' intimate knowledge of their area or from a local health promotion department or other external influence. These variable influences deserve some consideration.

There have been a number of government policy documents on health promotion and the *Health of the Nation* White Paper outlined a policy focus on a limited number of areas of priority action, including coronary heart disease, mental health and cancer (DoH 1992). These government targets were later endorsed in the two White Papers (DoH 1999, SODoH 1999) and adopted in turn by health boards and health authorities, as purchasers, and as a consequence community trusts had to respond as providers. As Stone (1996) has argued, government targets have also engendered a spate of activity within health promotion departments who may also act as a resource for and an influence over health-visiting activity. Health visitor health promotion activity at the level of the population has to remain sensitive to such targets and may benefit from the prioritising decisions which this will confer. Clearly, a wide range of traditional health-visiting interventions such as weight reduction, anti-smoking and healthy lifestyle programmes which are undertaken in groups and schools can be fitted easily within the ambit of such targets. However, community profiles and the evidence collected in the course of day-to-day work will inevitably identify other important areas such as post-natal and parenting support and child safety initiatives. The ability of health visitors to respond to such issues must be encouraged in order to meet government requirements that services be sensitive to local needs (DHSS 1989).

However, given a climate of resource constraint and limited time, there is potential for conflict between the interventions which are linked to government targets for health promotion and interventions designed to meet other, more locally defined needs. There is the additional factor of the health improvement programmes to be pursued by primary care groups, primary care trusts and local health-care cooperatives in Scotland and the influence which these may have on the health promotion and public health activity of health visitors (DoH 1997, SODoH 1997). As Young & Haynes (1993) have argued, the dispersed nature of many GP practices is not the ideal basis upon which to assess or address the needs of a population. There is as yet insufficient evidence to determine how these organisational arrangements within primary care will affect the work of health visitors but one point is certain: the GP's practice as a unit of health promotion activity may be inefficient in terms of the wider public health remit and health visitors will have to remain vigilant about the ways in which this aspect of their public health role may be influenced.

While it has been effectively argued that health visitors lack a framework of needs assessment, it is also the case that they are not free agents in terms of developing their public health role. Rather, they are constrained by a range of competing influences and sources of power. While a significant proportion of their work remains child centred with needs assessment operating at the individual level, their public health role is shaped by national targets mediated by health authorities/health boards, primary care groups, primary care trusts, health promotion departments and by local health-care cooperatives in Scotland (DoH 1997, SODoH 1997). As noted earlier, it could now be argued that policy directives on strengthening the public health function and targeting inequality appear to provide a strong case for community development approaches to achieving better health for the population (DoH 1999, SODoH 1999).

The strong government endorsement of the 'new public health' together with the introduction of health authority/health board health improvement programmes raise key questions about the ways in which need for health visiting interventions in the public health field will be identified. At the time of writing, there are no clear indications as to how this may be pursued except that the responsibility for assessing need is placed firmly with the health authorities/health boards. It has to be recognised that the needs assessment activities undertaken by health authorities/boards may be broad brush and disease oriented; therefore there may still be considerable scope for health visiting to influence the strategies for identifying and meeting need. This will represent a considerable challenge, because of the necessity of including the 'softer, more qualitative data' referred to earlier and also because of the specific demands which the adoption of a community development approach could bring (Cowley & Billings 1999).

For example, greater attention needs to be given to the 'verifiable states' which health visitors are required to address and the mechanisms by which these can be prioritised. While the structure of needs assessment proposed by Liss refers to the value-laden nature of decisions regarding goals and the means of reaching the goals, it may also be necessary to acknowledge that the 'verifiable states' themselves may not readily be decided by traditional 'objective' means such as epidemiological data or other statistics. Moreover, if a community development model is espoused, then the 'verifiable states', goals and means of achieving the goals may be heavily influenced by members of the public. As a consequence, health visitors may experience a tension between working to this agenda while at the same time maintaining links with health improvement programmes.

District nursing

While district nurses are not generally regarded as having to fulfil a dual role in the way that health visitors are, there is an important public health dimension of needs assessment in their work which is seldom acknowledged. While some patients and clients have health-care needs which could be described as 'single state' in the sense that there is a single problem or need to be addressed such as a varicose ulcer, many others will have a number of interrelated health needs each of which requires a goal and a means of reaching the goal. This could apply, for example, to an elderly person with multiple pathology. In such cases, while it may be possible to establish a factual basis for a series of needs or states, it may be difficult to set goals or develop a realistic plan for achieving all the goals. Practitioners may find they have to adapt goals, make compromises in the course of their plans or set priorities for intervention where some goals have to be temporarily set aside.

There are therefore identifiable additional stages in the needs assessment process which have not always been recognised by writers in the field but which appear to be related to the presence of complex needs. Complexity of need is a manifestation of the shift from hospital to community care, the ageing of the population, the association of poverty with ill health and changes in technology which allow greater degrees of medical intervention. The assessment of complex need involves processes which are poorly understood because district nurses themselves have not focused on them in depth in the course of professional discussion and there has been insufficient research effort in the field to assist understanding (Bryans & McIntosh 1996). There is an important public health dimension to this difficulty.

It could be argued that the assessment of complex need and the prioritising decisions which are associated with it are difficult to translate to a population level. The level and nature of community nursing intervention can potentially vary quite widely for patients and clients with ostensibly the same conditions because of the contextual influences referred to above, together with the patients' or clients' variable views about the level of intervention they are prepared to accept. For this reason, practitioners understand implicitly that investigating the incidence of particular health problems such as cerebrovascular accidents in the population will not offer a logical basis for addressing individual needs. Indeed, for reasons of individual and contextual variation, it may appear that there is a major discontinuity between assessment of individual need and assessment of need at the population level. This is a serious issue given the expectation that community nurses will fulfil a public health role with its connotations of understanding the health needs of the population.

In the first place, district nurses have fewer benchmarks, such as the birth rate, by which to assess the overall population need for their intervention. There are very few population or community-based investigations, epidemiological or otherwise, which offer a sound basis for establishing what the need for district nursing intervention will be. It could be argued that this will reduce the confidence which district nurses have in initiatives designed to assess the health needs of the communities in which they work. However, there is an important reason why district nurses need to consider the overall needs of the population. In the process of their prioritising decisions, it is possible that certain aspects of care for some patients have to be delayed or undertaken in a less intensive way in the interests of other patients with more serious conditions or more urgent needs. As the effects of these decisions are compounded across a particular population, certain needs may not be addressed, for example those experienced by the overstretched carer or the less obvious health needs of the frail elderly who now have to rely on social services/work departments to minister to their personal and other care. The sum total of these prioritising decisions may amount to a considerable deficit in public health which is unknown and difficult, if not impossible, to appraise.

There is no apparent health board or health authority strategy for prioritising district nursing care in the area of complex needs and with the requirements for strict financial control which have been imposed on trusts, community nurse managers have a reduced ability to manage resources in a locally sensitive way in order to address such problems. Lastly, the current systems of recording district nursing activity are not conducive to an appraisal of prioritising decisions. Such problems are, of course, not unique to district nursing. The same arguments about complex needs frequently confront health visitors in their care of families living in deprived circumstances.

METHODS OF POPULATION NEEDS ASSESSMENT

Community nurses are urged from within the profession to develop more proactive and broader approaches to needs assessment, taking account of the needs of the populations they serve, and in particular to contribute to the central public health issues of the day (SNMAC 1995). In addition, health authorities and health boards are charged with the responsibility for assessing the health needs of the population in order to inform the commissioning process. Community nurses contribute to such exercises by the collection of statistics on their work, by caseload profiling and by informal initiatives within and between their practice bases. However, there is no evidence of mechanisms set up to facilitate the sharing of such data and no structures other than the commissioning process by which agreement on the nature and extent of need can be achieved. In relation to the identification of need at the level of the population, there are no guidelines or principles laid down and no requirements laid upon the different groups, such as specialists in public health medicine, health promotion, health visitors and GPs, to work collaboratively on priorities.

Clearly, a framework which incorporates needs assessment at both an individual and a community or population level ought to be a prerequisite for effective practice. It is not clear from the literature on needs assessment whether such a framework exists and evidence from a recent research study conducted by the author and others suggests that there are a number of barriers in formulating one (Worth et al 1995, Carney et al 1996, Lugton et al 1998).

The research study was conducted in several health centres and community mental health resource centres in a large Scottish city with a population of 750 000 people. The methods, which have been described in detail elsewhere, included documenting referrals to three different community nursing groups: district nurses, health visitors and community psychiatric nurses (Worth et al 1995, Carney et al 1996, Lugton et al 1998). It also involved a small-scale survey of target groups which normally formed an important element of the caseloads of the three groups in an effort to identify whether there was unmet need. Finally, the study included in-depth interviews with practitioners, GPs and social workers.

One of the strands running through all three stages of the study was the extent to which the three groups identified need at the level of their community or population. One of the research objectives was to identify whether there was evidence that community health profiles were used and if so, how the results of such investigations were built into practice. The study sample comprised 20 district nurses, 16 health visitors and 16 community psychiatric nurses working in a total of five different locations. The district nurse group was asked about their use of community health profiles and their value as a means of identifying need. Only three out of the 20 had access to such profiles although the majority (12) said that profiles would be helpful in familiarising themselves with local resources and as a means of teaching students about the neighbourhood. Only five of the district nurses noted the value of the community health profile as a tool for 'identifying needs and planning of services to meet need' (Worth et al 1995, p. 72). However, the district nurses reported that they lacked the time required for the development and maintenance of a community profile. As far as the health visitor sample was concerned, 14 out of the 16 stated that they did not use community health profiles and had not been involved in their compilation. However, two health visitors who acted as community practice teachers did use profiles but mainly as a teaching tool rather than as a guide to practice.

Given the explicit public health role of the health visitor, this lack of the use of profiles was surprising because there was evidence of a considerable amount of group work among practitioners. So the issue was pursued in order to find out whether they used any alternative sources of information in order to help them meet the public health needs of the population. It is noteworthy that 10 practitioners did use other strategies for identifying population needs and these included 'health board statistics, data gathered from locally run groups such as lifestyle clinics and census data' (Carney et al 1996, p. 54). Despite this positive use of material for the assessment of need at a population level, the overwhelming pattern of need identification within this group was at the level of the individual and there was no evidence of a coherent approach to the identification of need at the community level as a means of supporting or challenging the move made, at the time of the study, to refocus the health visitor role towards the elderly and the physically disabled.

BARRIERS TO POPULATION-BASED NEED IDENTIFICATION

Given the issues outlined above, the question of whether assessment of need at the level of the population is encouraged by GPs, providers or commissioners has to be addressed. There is no evidence to suggest that this is the case. Contracts for community nursing services are usually block contracts based on the activity levels of the previous year with the possibility of some modest adjustments made for any anticipated change. This approach may be a workable solution to the problem of achieving realistic contractual agreements but it is not conducive to proper appraisal of the health needs of the population. Health visitors are not in a position to defend their focus on children and mothers because there is a lack of data about the opportunity cost of refocusing health-visiting intervention elsewhere.

There appear to be few mechanisms for a proper interaction between the concern with the individual patient or client and the approach to needs assessment by the purchaser/commissioner. The process of needs assessment has not been subject to critical appraisal and community nurses have been criticised for an apparent lack of a framework. However, one of the problematic aspects of community practice is the variety of different contexts in which nurses give care and the way in which they have to adapt to individuals. Part of their expertise lies in such adaptation and thus variability of approach is arguably appropriate. In focusing on need at an individual level and in attempting to address the daily uncertainties within available resources, it is not surprising that few practitioners have worked out strategies for addressing population needs. The individual and idiosyncratic needs of clients on the caseload do not readily translate to the level of the population. Yet, as has been argued, in responding to a multiplicity of need and prioritising, community nurses are, by default, influencing the ways in which they meet the needs of the population as a whole.

Can the strategies for addressing complex need be formulated at the level of a community or a population in such a way as to inform and guide practice, the shape of the service or the use of resources? An explanation of how such a macro view should inform community nursing practice is required. It is difficult for community nurses themselves to adopt such an approach because they lack control over information systems and therefore have no basis from which to argue a case. They also lack direct access to expert advice from statisticians and economists and so are in a weak position vis-à-vis managers who are able to call upon such resources. Yet, as has been shown, managers have attempted to refocus both the health visitor and the district nurse role without recourse to evidence or a rationale for change. Thus, it is likely that issues of equity and redistribution within and between communities are fraught with political sensitivity, organisational barriers and practical problems in terms of introducing change.

An additional problem stems from the fact that a population approach would need to gain agreement from the entire primary health-care team, commissioners and other influential groups in the field. Such an approach would therefore require community nurses to build and maintain alliances with a number of different interest groups. Given that such groups are likely to be operating from different models of public health, this is not a straightforward process.

In conclusion, it appears that with regard to assessing the needs of the population and providing the basis for a coherent range of activity at that level, practitioners experience a considerable array of problems. Philosophical and theoretical discussions of the concept of need, while useful in some respects, are not sufficiently broad to encompass the prioritising decisions which have to be made between needs experienced by the same individual or the same group or to fully account for the influence of context. Is it possible to identify a way forward? One possible solution may lie within the field of community development approaches to assessing need and promoting action for health, as discussed in Chapter 8.

DISCUSSION

Public health can be interpreted as including not only the maintenance of health by means of health education, health promotion and various strategies of prevention but also achieving the best possible mental and physical well-being of those who are sick or disabled and those who care for them. In this wider sense, all community nurses have a contribution to make to public health and this chapter has argued that they should understand the intricacies of assessing the needs of the populations which they serve.

At the most basic level, a population-based assessment of need helps to define the social, economic and epidemiological attributes of a community. While it may have been assumed in the past that such a profile would offer an indication of the services which might need to be provided, a number of approaches to such information could be adopted. It is important to make more explicit the links between the findings of such a profile and the social conditions which influence health. Such an approach might significantly change the strategies used to promote health, involving, for example, community development initiatives as described in Chapter 8 rather than initiatives targeted at the level of small groups.

While much of community nursing activity takes place at the level of the individual, it is essential to acknowledge the reasons why assessment of need at the level of the population is important. If there is a lack of clarity about such reasons, it is all too easy to focus all effort at the individual level because this is where the immediate or obvious health-care needs are presented. Population-based assessment of need should be undertaken in order to address issues of equity and distribution as well as to provide an optimum basis for planning services. There is also a further key factor which deserves critical appraisal and that is the impact, however slow, of demographic or technological change. Population projections are fraught with difficulty but if there is strong evidence of growth or decline within certain vulnerable groups within the population then community nurses should seek ways of providing evidence of the impact of such change upon their activity. Given that community nurses are making prioritising decisions throughout their work, an understanding of need at the level of the population should encourage a more critical interrogation of practice and enable practitioners to appraise their rationales for decisions made at the individual level within the framework of a wider viewpoint.

Health visitors operate very successfully at the level of the small group for the communities within which they work and to this extent identifying and addressing need has moved beyond the level of the individual. However, while the merits of such initiatives are not in doubt, many of them may be ad hoc and confined to a neighbourhood. They may succumb to reductions in staffing and have a precarious financial foundation. They therefore do not necessarily provide a sufficient basis for demonstrating the value of professional input, they are not conducive to promoting a theoretical framework for intervention and they are unlikely to achieve the critical mass required for support and commitment from other health-care colleagues. It could be argued that a population-based needs assessment, as a precursor to such group work, would render such activity more focused. It might involve uncomfortable choices but a more extensive concentration on selected areas of health promotion might resolve some of the problems of diffuse activity, lack of frameworks and the challenges of measuring outcomes.

In the recent past, the purchaser/provider split meant that health boards and health authorities, as purchasers, tried to extract as much value as possible from the contracts which they agreed with trusts. At the same time, as part of their role in the contracting process, trusts attempted to retain business by offering good value for money. It was therefore in the interests of neither to address needs in a systematic way. Caught in a contractual and financial relationship which set them apart, rather than binding them together, the two groups which previously could form a powerful alliance in promoting the health interest of the population were rendered less able to create the framework within which health-care professionals can identify population needs and develop strategies for meeting them. The dissipation of the internal market in health care, together with the positive endorsement of cross-sectoral working in both White Papers (DoH 1999, SoDoH 1999), ought to make a significant contribution to reversing this process. In the short term, it appears that an alliance among professional groups, while presenting some difficulties and challenges, is the only way forward in an effort to develop a coherent and sensitive framework in which both individual and population health-care needs can be addressed and met. It is to be hoped that commissioning by GPs and community nurses working together in PCGs and local health-care cooperatives will be more conducive to a broader view of need and public health priorities.

However, community nurses may also need to develop their systems for analysing health needs in quite different ways. Health visitors require a broad view of the health needs of their communities and this may help to target interventions at both the individual and the population level. For example, if the rate of pregnancy among single teenage girls is rising, health visitors could target individual attention upon this group of clients to ensure that they had sufficient support for the development of parenting skills. In addition, though, they may also aim health promotion initiatives at school or youth groups. As Cowley (1997) has pointed out, they need to work seamlessly between individual, family and community. This population assessment would therefore mean work at both the individual and group levels. On the other hand, district nurses seldom work at the group level and an understanding of population health needs would inform practice in a different way. For example, knowledge of ward closures or an increase in early discharge and an understanding of the way in which other local policies influence the provision for ill people are key features of developing strategies to ensure that health need is properly addressed.

CONCLUSION

This chapter has attempted to show some of the challenges involved in assessing individual and population-based health-care needs and the ways in which certain difficulties can foster disagreement about the role of community nurses in public health. It has been argued that an attempt by nurses to analyse needs at the level of the population and a subsequent prioritising of intervention could lay a strong foundation for testing existing needs assessment models, such as that proposed by Liss, or for evolving new models. A more concerted and collaborative approach to the assessment of need would require alliances with other groups of health-care professionals but this could provide opportunities for addressing issues of equity and offer a clearer picture of the value of the nursing contribution to the health of individuals and the population.

REFERENCES

Badger F, Cameron E, Evers H 1988 Nursing in perspective. Health Service Journal 98(5127): 1362–1363

Bradshaw J 1972 A taxonomy of social need. In McLachlan G (ed) Problems and progress in medical care – essays in current research. Oxford University Press, Oxford, pp 71–82

Bryans A, McIntosh J 1998 Decision making in community nursing: an analysis of the stages of decision making as they relate to community nursing assessment practice. Journal of Advanced Nursing 24

Carney O, McIntosh J, Worth A, Lugton J 1996 Assessment of need for health visiting. Monograph No. 2, Caledonian University, Glasgow

Cernik K, Wearne M 1992 Using community health profiles to improve service provision. Health Visitor 65(10): 343–345

Cervi B 1993 Advice on unmet need a legal muddle, say SSDs. Community Care March: 6

Chalmers K 1993 Searching for health needs: the work of health visiting. Journal of Advanced Nursing 18: 900–911

Cowley S 1995 Health-as-process: a health visiting perspective. Journal of Advanced Nursing 22: 433–441

Cowley S 1997 Public health values in practice: the case of health visiting. Critical Public Health 7(1&2): 82–97

Cowley S, Billings J R 1999 Implementing new health visiting services through action research: an analysis of process. Journal of Advanced Nursing 30(4): 965–974

Craig P 1995 Health visiting and health promotion. Greater Glasgow Community and Mental Health Services NHS Trust, Glasgow (unpublished)

DHSS 1989 Caring for people: community care in the next decade and beyond. White Paper Cm 849. HMSO, London

DoH 1990 NHS and Community Care Act. HMSO, London

DoH 1992 The health of the nation – a strategy for England. Department of Health, London

DoH 1997 The new NHS: modern, dependable. Cm 3807. Stationery Office, London

DoH 1999 Saving lives. Our healthier nation. Cm 4386. Stationery Office, London

DoH/SSI 1991 Assessment systems and community care. Department of Health Social Services Inspectorate, London

Doyal L, Gough I 1991 A theory of human need. Macmillan, Basingstoke

Fatchett A B 1990 Health visiting: a withering profession? Journal of Advanced Nursing 15: 216–222

Griffiths R 1988 Community care – agenda for action. A report to the Secretary for State for the Social Services. HMSO, London

Hawtin M, Hughes G, Percy-Smith J 1994 Community profiling: auditing social needs. Open University Press, Buckingham

Liss P E 1993 Health care need – meaning and measurement. Ashgate Publishing, Avebury

Lugton J, McIntosh J, Carney O, Worth A 1998 Identifying need for community psychiatric nursing intervention. Research monograph No. 3. Glasgow Caledonian University, Glasgow

Luker K A, Orr J 1992 Health visiting. Blackwell, London

Luker K A, Perkins E S 1988 Lay carer's views of the district nursing service. Midwife, Health Visitor and Community Nurse 24(4): 132–134

McIntosh J, Lockhart K, Atkinson P, Fraser S, Lynch M 1994 A review of community nursing services in Glasgow. Caledonian University, Glasgow

McWalter G, Toner H, Corser A, Eastwood J, Marshall M, Turvey T 1994 Needs and needs assessment: their components and definitions with reference to dementia. Health and Social Care 2: 213–219

Murray S A, Graham L J C 1995 Practice based health needs assessment: use of four methods in a small neighbourhood. British Medical Journal 310: 1443–1448

Ong B N, Humphris G, Annett H, Rifkin S 1991 Rapid appraisal in an urban setting: an example from the developed world. Social Science and Medicine 32 (8): 909–915

Powell C 1995 Scoring for goals: identifying need among health visitor clients. Child Health 2(4): 155–159

Robinson J 1985 Health visiting and health. In: White R (ed) Political issues in nursing: past, present and future. John Wiley, Chichester

Schultz P R, Magilvy J K 1988 Assessing community health needs of elderly populations: comparisons of three strategies. Journal of Advanced Nursing 13 (2): 193–202

Scottish Office Department of Health 1997 Designed to care. Renewing the National Health Service in Scotland. Cm 3811. Stationery Office, Edinburgh

Scottish Office Department of Health 1999 Towards a healthier Scotland. Cm 4269. Stationery Office, Edinburgh

Seedhouse D 1994 Fortress NHS: a philosophical review of the National Health Service. John Wiley, Chichester

Shepherd M 1992 Comparing need with resource allocation. Health Visitor 65(9): 303–306

Smith G 1980 Social need policy: practice research. Routledge and Kegan Paul, London

Standing Nursing and Midwifery Advisory Committee 1995 Making it happen. Public health – the contribution, role and development of nurses, midwives and health visitors. Department of Health, London

Stone D 1996 Visiting time. Health Services Journal 106 (5497): 28–29

Thomas E 1997 Community nursing profiles: their role in needs assessment. Nursing Standard 11(37): 39–42

Twinn S 1991 Conflicting paradigms of health visiting: a continuous debate for professional practice. Journal of Advanced Nursing 16 (8): 966–973

Twinn S, Dauncey J, Carnell J 1990 The process of health profiling. Health Visitors' Association, London

Worth A, McIntosh J, Carney O, Lugton J 1995 Assessment of need for district nursing. Monograph No. 1. Glasgow Caledonian University, Glasgow

Young K, Haynes R 1993 Assessing population needs in primary health care: the problem of GP attachment. Journal of Interprofessional Care 7(1): 15–27

8

Community development as a strategy for public health

Yvonne Dalziel

INTRODUCTION

Community development models have been applied to health issues and health care since the self-help and women's health movements of the early 1970s. This chapter describes the growth of community development models within health and demonstrates that key concepts in community development and the methods used to effect the challenges of the 1960s and 1970s were a reaction to dominant societal systems. The chapter explores how the principles of community development offer nurses a method of working with public health issues and suggests that these concepts, methods and approaches are pertinent to the execution of public health nursing today.

DEFINITIONS

Public health is defined as 'the science and art of preventing disease, prolonging life and promoting health through organised efforts of society'

(Acheson 1988). The aim of public health is to improve the health of communities by providing protection from environmental hazards and responding to health needs (Watkins 1994). Therefore, public health not only addresses social and environmental causes of ill health but also seeks to improve the health of neighbourhoods.

A similar definition is suggested by SNMAC (1995) for *public health in nursing*:

... public health in nursing, midwifery and health visiting practice is about commissioning health services and providing professional care through organised collaboration in the NHS and society, to protect and promote health and well-being, prolong life and prevent ill-health in local communities groups and populations'.

The emphasis is on protection and the prevention of harm to communities and nurses are viewed as having a key role in this activity.

Community appears to be a simple concept often used as a blanket term to describe a geographical population. In reality, it is a fairly complex notion. It can mean a group of people who live in the same street, same village or same town but it can also describe a number of individuals with something in common who may or may not acknowledge that connection. The latter are often called communities of interest and can include groups such as ethnic minorities, pensioners, people with AIDS or deaf women. Iscoe (1974) proposed that the purpose of community work is to build a 'competent community', by which he meant one that can 'care for its members and help them to cope with or to change external forces'.

However, the notion that communities, including communities of interest, are homogeneous collections of like-minded people with similar interests is misleading. Communities, however defined, can be riven with conflict: the needs of the young against the needs of the old, men and women, able and disabled, black and white.

Hawe (1994) suggests that a competent community would be one that is able to tackle the problems which beset it through harnessing its internal resources: collective experiences, skills and energy as well as external resources for community-determined solutions.

Community development in health is said to:

... encompass a commitment to a holistic approach to health which recognises the central importance of social support and social networks. A community way of working attempts to facilitate individual and collective action around common needs and concerns identified by the community itself and not imposed from outside. (OU/HEA 1990)

The emphasis is on working collaboratively to address equity, support democracy and the participation of the community in issues that affect their lives.

Although community development is now gaining recognition as an approach to improving health, the methods and thinking that constitute community development are not new. Jones (1990) suggests that it was used by colonial governments to 'ensure the governability and modernisation of their empires' (p. 32). It was more recent events, however, that nurtured its growth and its value as an approach to addressing health issues.

INFLUENCES OF SOCIAL MOVEMENTS ON COMMUNITY DEVELOPMENT IN HEALTH

According to Jones (1990), 'Community development and health work has evolved over the last ten years, incorporating a number of different influences which have built onto a basic community development model'. The growing movement in health occurring in the last few decades has used community development as an ideological and practical framework to change the way in which health is regarded as a concept. Previously used as a method in community work to address housing and social policy needs, the first health projects using community development principles of participation and partnership did not appear in the UK until the late 1970s. The emergence of social movements like the women's movement, civil rights, black power and the self-help movement were key influences in supporting the growth of the approach.

A social movement is defined as: 'collectivity acting with some continuity to promote change in the society or group to which it is a part' (Turner & Killian quoted in Schiller & Levin 1983, p. 1344). The social movements of the 1960s and 1970s grew from the disaffection of people who felt marginal to and excluded from decision-making processes. They were a reaction to the dominant male, white middle-class systems and the attitudes that discriminated against women, black people and the poor. The movements demanded justice, freedom, democracy and the end of discrimination. Underpinning their emergence was a belief system that held primacy of individual experience as the basis of knowledge and expertise.

The primary challenge of both the women's health movement (which grew out of the women's liberation movement) and the self-help movement was to the mystification and ownership of knowledge by the male-dominated medical profession. There developed at that time an antiprofessional view of health and the causes of ill health. Individuals were encouraged to become experts on their own bodies and to view what they knew, derived from their own experiences, as being as important as the theoretical knowledge evolved conceptually and filtered through a dominant male medical ideology. This was an ideology that viewed women as somehow feebler in mind and body, prone to being emotional, unable to manage their own affairs and being unsuitable for responsibilities outwith the home. In consciousness-raising groups and in self-help health groups, women began to see how this view of themselves was reinforced by their contact with the medical profession and that it adversely affected their health and their access to health services.

The essential message of the social movements was that the poor and disadvantaged, both socially and economically, were experts on their own lives with knowledge and experience that could be used to promote and sustain healthy communities. The seminal Black Report (Townsend & Davidson 1983) indicated that it is these groups who are more likely to experience poorer health and have shorter lives than more affluent people.

The Alma-Ata declaration of 1978 states that 'The people have a right and a duty to participate individually and collectively in the planning and implementation of their care'. The desire for a public health movement to tackle health problems resulted in 1981 in the WHO policy of Health for All by the year 2000. Central to the attainment of its targets is the development of primary care and the concepts of participation, collaboration and equity that were central to the Alma-Ata declaration.

The key tenets of a community development approach, i.e. collectivity, self-determination, democracy and promotion of self-confidence, are central to any policy to tackle inequalities in health. The gap that exists in public health knowledge about the needs of the poorest communities could be addressed by a community development public health strategy. This would legitimate the approach and support the move away from the clinical model based on individual transactions to a social contract with entire communities (Ashton & Seymour 1988).

ELEMENTS OF COMMUNITY DEVELOPMENT

A community development approach is therefore a useful way to move from exclusion to inclusion in the decision-making process for marginal groups. The principles which underpin the approach and make the invisible visible are as follows.

- Equity
- Empowerment
- Participation
- Cooperation and collaboration
- Partnership and alliances
- Community-led needs assessment

Equity

This is the belief that people should have equal access to available services for the maintenance and promotion of health and where none exist, they should be provided. It seeks to eradicate inequalities in the experience of health, not only in the provision of services but in the methods of service delivery. It challenges practices that discriminate against individuals on whatever basis: colour, disability, language, sexuality or age.

Empowerment

Rappaport et al define empowerment as 'the process by which people, organisations and communities gain mastery over their lives' (1984, p. 3). The empowerment process involves building individual and collective confidence and raising the esteem of individuals and communities, through valuing their knowledge and experience and supporting them to be part of the decision-making process. Kiefer (1983), quoted in Meleis (1992), views empowerment as attainment of what he calls 'participatory competence'. Beigal (1984) views empowerment as both capacity and equity, capacity being use of power to solve problems and equity referring to getting one's fair share of resources. Empowerment skills include problem solving, assertiveness and confidence-building strategies.

Participation

Participation is about supporting people affected by decisions to have some influence over their outcome. Involving people as part of the decision-making process is beneficial not only to those living in communities but also to the service providers. Giving users a say in what they need avoids the mismatch of services and may in the long run be more economical.

Perception of power affects participation. Steve Lukes (1978) suggests that there are different levels of power: the visible manifestations of power, the unseen but tangible manifestations of power and internalised powerlessness. People on the margins of society often experience this third level of powerlessness and become passive. Believing they cannot influence events and decisions affecting their lives, they exclude themselves from opportunities to be part of the process of decision making. Kiefer (1983) suggests that participatory competence is a lifelong achievement and includes three aspects:

1. development of a more positive self-concept or sense of self-competence;
2. construction of more critical or analytical understanding of the surrounding social and political environment;
3. cultivation of individual and collective resources for social and political action.

Consultation rather than participation happens when decisions have already been made and there is little likelihood of any change but the public is still asked to comment about a proposal. This is a poor substitute for real participation and being part of the planning process.

Partnership and alliances

A key concept in the community development process is partnership and the building of alliances. An alliance is defined as a partnership for action, a virtual organisation created by the interaction between partner agencies and sectors (Duffy 1996). The purpose of agencies working together and with local people is to develop common priorities and strategies on issues and policies that affect health. Partnerships for health involve a wider spectrum than is usually associated with the health sector. For example, a health alliance would involve nurses working in partnership with agencies such as environmental health, education, social work, voluntary organisations, health projects, workplaces and local industries.

There are five key features of alliance building (Funnel et al 1995):

1. *commitment* – a shared commitment to the goals of the alliance. Participants have the necessary skills and members give what resources they can;
2. *community involvement* – partnership with the community in all alliance activities. Community representatives have the necessary training and skills to participate equally;
3. *communication* – partners share relevant information and commit to simplicity, openness and honesty;
4. *joint working* – implies equal ownership and appropriate input from each partner;
5. *accountability* – evaluation is built into alliance work and results used constructively.

The benefits of community partnerships to nurses in relation to pooling information, knowledge, experience, skills and resources are substantial. Joint working can be more efficient and effective and can widen and deepen the impact of health initiatives. In return, nurses must be willing to share knowledge with communities and to be involved in training and supporting community involvement.

Community-led needs assessment

A popular epidemiological approach to assessing need is to view people as population groups on a national grid differentiated by social class, age or geographical location. However neat this may be as a way of determining trends and assessing need in populations, it nevertheless ignores the fact that people largely draw the values, interests and concerns that influence their health choices and the way they live their lives from the dominant culture of the community in which they live; either their geographical neighbourhood or the perceived community of interest to which they feel they belong. People living in a culture with shared values can, however, have different access to services, e.g. rural and inner city or peripheral housing estates, and people living in specific geographical communities do not necessarily share similar needs and aspirations with the rest of the community and may have needs that are in conflict. Given the complexity of the influences on health, the process of finding out what individuals, communities or populations need to support or promote health is very complicated.

'Not all human experience is measurable in numbers and that which is not may be more important than that which is', according to Watkins (1994). The 1990 NHS and Community Care Act moved some of the way to recognising that if services are set up in isolation from the people who use them, they may not meet their needs, leading to inappropriate or patchy use. The implementation of the Act meant that health and social services in the community were required to work more closely with the people who live in the areas they serve. However, health needs assessment has been largely professionally driven, derived from what is available and manageable, with solutions to identified need often located within the medical arena. On the other hand, community development is about helping communities define their own needs and then be part of the process of meeting these needs. In this way, services can be developed in a more relevant and appropriate manner.

The following section explores the potential for health visitors to embrace a community development approach and to begin to adapt and learn new skills so that concepts such as empowerment, equity, participation and collaboration become meaningful and contribute to public health policy. The considerable structural barriers to working in this way are also discussed.

ESTABLISHING A ROLE FOR NURSES IN COMMUNITY DEVELOPMENT

The recognition of widening inequality in access to health and health-care services is creating increasing pressure on the primary care team. If community development approaches can help communities be involved in holistically addressing the issues they identify as barriers to health, primary care nurses may need to change the focus of their work away from individual illness models to support communities to collectively promote public health in their area. Health visitors are well placed to take a lead in a more community-orientated approach for the following reasons.

- Community development principles match the principles of health visiting.
- Health visitors are already working in public health promotion in the community.
- The remit for health visiting is changing.
- It is an interesting and challenging way to work which uses and develops existing health-visiting skills.

Principles of health visiting

The practice of health visiting is based on four principles:

1. the search for health needs;
2. stimulating the awareness of health needs;
3. encouraging health-enhancing activities;
4. influencing policies affecting health.

Given the definition of public health as encompassing protection and prevention, these are appropriate principles for a public health perspective on health. They are also, in the main, congruent with a community development approach.

Health visiting and community development share similar aims in their approaches to health. They both:

- promote an interest in and an understanding of positive health and well-being as defined by the WHO (1977);
- use definitions that encompass health in its widest sense;
- adopt a holistic and dynamic approach to health;
- view the recognition and fulfilment of need as primary objectives;
- share a belief in helping individuals use their own resources to overcome difficulties;
- help create access to health resources and information about health.

One of four principles central to the practice of health visiting focuses on influencing policy. However, health visitors have not been noted in the past for their contribution to policies affecting health or for their challenge to policies that do nothing to eliminate causes of ill health. As field workers within the present structures, it is difficult for them to access the policy-making process. Working with community development methods offers health visitors a role in developing health policies at a local level that fulfils the scope of the principles (Craig 1998).

Health visitors already working in the community

Health visitors are presently in the community working with people most at risk and whose voices are least represented in the policy-making processes: women with children, young people, older people, unemployed, disabled and other disadvantaged groups such as homeless and travellers. They know first hand what affects people. They know that poverty, unemployment, high crime rates and poor housing have a direct impact on health in a community. They know that the experience of poverty creates low self-confidence and stops individuals and groups of people participating in educational opportunities for growth and self-improvement. They know that lack of money leads to poor diets and low energy, that lack of services and counselling keeps people tied to old patterns of behaviour that do not support their health and well-being. They know that they do 'crisis visits' which may do little to change the underlying issues because there is no one else to offer families in chaotic situations the support they need. They know, along with others in primary care, that as individual workers they are trying to meet community and individual needs without the appropriate structures or services to support them. It is argued that integrating a community development approach into mainstream work is an opportunity for the profession to create the services and structures they need to address the difficulties they face daily in trying to meet community health need.

Changing remit for health visitors

The impact of commissioning and the development of a market economy in health resulted in health-visiting services being viewed by some as lacking evidence of effectiveness and efficiency within the parameters of medical interventions. Much of health visitors' work remains invisible because it takes place in private. Community development approaches within a public health agenda, rather than working in isolation, would make health-visiting practice more visible. Although community development activity can be as difficult to evaluate scientifically as health visiting, the impact in a community is more easily audited qualitatively and through process measures.

Uses existing health-visiting knowledge and skills

Health visitors may not have all the necessary skills and knowledge to work collectively and in participation with communities but their grounding as community health workers is something on which to build. With extra training and support, they could potentially undertake different health-promoting activities. This theme is explored further in the following section.

CONSTRAINTS ON HEALTH VISITORS USING A COMMUNITY DEVELOPMENT APPROACH

Health visitors have the potential to work with community development approaches within neighbourhoods and with communities of interest. Despite this potential, a small study undertaken by the author (Dalziel 1997) of health visitors undergoing community development training shows that the following factors militate against health visitors as community development workers:

- the assumption that health visitors are primarily caseload workers;
- their location as part of the primary care team in medical centres;
- lack of support, including training, management support and resources.

Focus on caseload work

Historically, health visitors were primarily public health nurses preventing illness by working with population groups. In recent times, however, they have been viewed more as caseload workers with the under-5s and the elderly, population groups that are perceived traditionally as the most vulnerable in the community. Currently, training and management support, not surprisingly, is geared to fulfilling this caseload remit. The concentration on an individual approach with families leaves little time for health visitors to work with population groups who are arguably more 'vulnerable' to ill health than the under-5s, and the elderly living in affluent communities, such as the homeless, travellers and people living in areas of economic deprivation.

There is some evidence from local studies that a community development approach can be viewed as 'icing on the cake' by health visitors (Dalziel 1997, White 1998). In the study mentioned above (Dalziel 1997), health visitors liked working in this way and believed it to be relevant to the promotion of health but felt constrained in practice by having a caseload. One health visitor who had completed community development training said, 'The main problem is finding the time away from the caseload to participate and put into practice what I learned'. Another barrier identified was the location of health visitors within primary care teams. 'I would like the other members of the primary care team to be aware of the principles (of community development) and for us to work together to improve the area we work in.'

Location of health visitors in primary care teams

Ideologically, most health visitors work with a social model of health but increasingly, their location within health centres and GP practices as part of the primary care team must pull them away from the communities in which they work and direct them more towards medical concerns. The essential differences in the medical and social models of health are located within authority and power issues, as illustrated in Box 8.1.

The essential differences between the medical and social models of health lie in how each views participation and partnership. The increasing demands on GPs for medical solutions to what are essentially social problems indicate that the medicalisation of private life is very potent. Sarason (1974) argues that the creation and maintenance of a sense of community could act as an antidote to the hopelessness and alienation of modern life. The role of the public health nurse working with a social model approach might be to help the community return to that sense of harnessing its own strengths and creating its own solutions that it has lost.

Box 8.1   Comparing medical and social models of health

Medical model	Social model
Works with an individual perspective	Works collectively to harness group knowledge and strength
The health agenda is set by professionals and their skills and knowledge are paramount	Values lay experience and knowledge and creates joint agendas with the community
The body is seen as a machine	Views social conditions as affecting health
No emphasis on participation	Brings people together to seek collective solutions
Concerned with numbers and quantitative methods	Values people's experience
Knowledge is guarded	Knowledge is shared
Looks for measurable outcomes	Values process as much as outcomes
No intersectoral collaboration	Looks for partnership and alliances

---

Lack of support: management, training and funding issues

Health visitors potentially have a key function in public health strategies and in regenerating communities despite health-visiting training currently being geared towards the support of individual families and not a community focus. From the study above, the lack of appropriate training, support from managers and resources to do the work (including adequate time) also emerged as substantial barriers to health visitors working in this way. Comments included, 'I haven't started community development work as I am not sure my manager would back me at the expense of my caseload'. Another health visitor, commenting on lack of managerial support, said, 'Management is not fully aware of the requirements/support involved and consequently can be unhelpful due to lack of understanding or non-commitment'.

RESTRUCTURING THE HEALTH VISITOR ROLE

It is only arguably in the current century that small communities began to lose the self-supporting functions that have now been replaced by professionals. Members of communities counselled the distressed, nursed the ill, delivered babies, doctored using natural remedies, guided, policed and acted as advocates for their members. They had what Sarason calls the psychological sense of community – the sense of belonging and shared ties that adds meaning and perspective to life. Health visitors have demonstrated that they have a role to play in recreating some of the self-supporting functions of communities in order to tackle the detrimental effects of material deprivation on health. As noted above, to be effective they would need their organisation to offer management support, appropriate resources and time. In addition, there would have to be the establishment of new working structures as well as the acquisition of new skills, knowledge and values.

Establishing new structures for working

In order to accommodate a new approach to health in nursing, a structure that allowed community development approaches to grow and evolve would need to be developed. One model proposed is that each health-visiting/primary care team or group of practices has designated health visitors employed to work with the following groups:

- the community, to help the process of articulation and meeting of health need;
- other allied workers in the community (housing, environmental health, education, etc.);
- mainstream health visitors and others in the team to develop a community-, as opposed to a practice-, orientated approach to health need.

Health visitors working with this approach would apply a community development approach to their own situation so that the work is under-pinned by principles of:

- working in partnership with other health visitor colleagues;
- alliance building with activists and others;
- collaboration with other agencies and local projects;
- collectivity, i.e. working as a group.

The designated health visitors would also work within the structures that already exist in the community, such as:

- community health projects;
- established projects working with issues of interest: food coops, children's projects, women's projects, homeless, etc.;
- groups in the community, e.g. women's groups, drug projects, educational groups, mothers and toddlers.

Acquisition of new knowledge and skills

Health visitors often express interest in a more community-oriented way of working but many believe that they do not have enough of the skills and knowledge needed to do this work. However, with appropriate training and/or support some health visitors around the UK have demonstrated that they can focus their work on the process of empowerment. Examples cited above described health visitors working with a social model of health where the community is encouraged to share common difficulties, knowledge and experience and to take collective action to bring about their own solutions.

Knowledge base for community development work

The body of knowledge that supports and helps the growth of community development includes the following:

* how agencies work and access to funding;
* local and community resources;
* knowledge of specific health issues, e.g. poverty, housing and health, men's and women's issues;
* how to access relevant information and materials for the community;
* methods of influencing policy;
* anti-discriminatory work;
* strategic planning.

Skills for community development work

Nurses arguably already have many of the skills needed for a community development approach including listening, counselling, organisation and management. However, they may need to learn others, such as:

* funding issues;
* awareness of the empowerment process;
* small group structures;
* needs assessment/community profiling;
* evaluation of community initiatives;
* alliance and partnership work;
* publicity and campaigning.

These skills in practice are discussed in greater detail in the following section.

Values of community development

There is an expectation that some of the values and qualities discussed here are already part of any nurse's value system. However, in the community, where practitioners are expected to work independently and there is little or no protection provided by the 'uniform', personal values are even more important.

Working with a community development approach demands that nurses work with people in a different way. The nature of the work requires a longer term, closer working relationship on a more equal basis than the traditional nurse/client/patient relationship and so demands different responses to support the work. Community development approaches are used to address socioeconomic inequalities and entail working with people with the least resources in our society. Not surprisingly, community members who become involved in community initiatives may suffer from low self-esteem and their educational and life experience leaves them doubting their own ability to achieve anything. They may also be reluctant to become involved for fear of being undermined and ridiculed for their efforts. In creating the right climate for participation, it is important for community members to trust the worker and know that he or she will respect their contribution, however small.

The success of community development work depends on involvement by the community. Basically, this is about how relationships between people are negotiated and managed. To work creatively and effectively in a community empowerment way, nurses must have an understanding of the following personal issues:

- awareness of personal authority and power issues;
- a clear understanding of personal and professional boundaries;
- awareness of own inner strengths and resources and the need for support;
- awareness of political ideologies;
- self-knowledge, e.g. own racist, sexist or other discriminatory feelings;
- commitment to equal opportunities;
- knowledge of personal limits and knowing when to let go.

COMMUNITY DEVELOPMENT ACTIVITY IN NURSING

Some of the activities nurses may be involved with in addressing public health issues as part of a community development remit include:

- helping communities identify their own needs, e.g. using community-orientated needs assessment and community profiling;
- mobilising neighbourhoods or communities of interest to harness their own skills and resources, e.g. setting up support groups, offering opportunities for volunteering or paid work;
- supporting people to get involved in their community and in decisions affecting their lives, e.g. offering training and supporting participation;
- engaging with the community in influencing policy, e.g. creating new structures and accessing existing structures for decision making;
- helping build healthy alliances between the community and people who can help them, e.g. sharing information, joint working.

Methods used may include small group structures and community profiling or needs assessment, described below.

Small group structures

Small groups are a useful method of working with a community development approach and are a common feature of community development work. The different kinds of group work with which nurses may be involved fall into several loose categories.

1. *Self-help groups or support groups*, e.g. menopause, depression, parents of special needs children. Pure self-help groups do exist in the community but more often groups are led by facilitators, usually community education workers and sometimes health visitors.

2. *Learning or training groups*, e.g. adult basic education, assertiveness training, volunteer training. Community workers and community activists use the small group structure as a method of getting people together to decide on a campaign or to set up a new service they have identified, e.g. a food coop or a women's group.

3. *Meeting/campaigning groups*, e.g. a health forum or an action group for a specific issue or campaign.

4. *Business groups*, e.g. management committees or steering groups.

Although these groups have a primary task they might also sometimes have a different function, e.g. a self-help group may become a campaign group around an issue and it may also be a learning group from time to time. A campaigning group will meet to do business but may also hold training sessions for its members. The main function of the facilitator or leader in these groups is to support the members to fulfil the group task. Ideally, the groups are democratic structures where the skill of the leader, worker or chairperson is to create an opportunity for as many people as possible to attend and for them to be able to participate fully.

The small group structure as a health-promoting method

The small group structure was an important element in the empowering process of the women's movement. Women came together in groups to share their experiences of health problems and to discover that collectively their wisdom was more relevant to their lives and health than much of the accepted knowledge of the medical profession. Together they campaigned to influence policies on women's issues such as abortion and contraception and on services that did not meet their needs. Maternity provision is a good example of a service provided by a statutory agency which has a history of leaving women feeling disempowered and demoralised.

The first Women's Health Fair was held in 1984 in Edinburgh and attracted wide publicity and much interest. Women's health groups began springing up from this time and although they initially attracted mainly white, middle-class women, the concept soon spread to other sections of society so that now they are a common feature of any community health activity. The small group structure offered women an opportunity to begin to discuss and develop an awareness of the wider issues around women's health such as mental health issues like depression, the use of prescribed drugs, sexuality and women's experience of violence.

Nurses as group facilitators

In order to work effectively with groups in the community, either in supporting their development or facilitating them as part of the empowerment process, health visitors need a high level of knowledge about group process, group dynamic and the skills to ensure that the group task is clear, manageable and that all members can contribute. Health visitors are generally involved in many groups in the community, e.g. mothers and toddlers and first-time mothers' groups, parentcraft sessions, dieting groups and sometimes carers' groups. These collective structures are often viewed as examples of community development. While group work is an important feature of the community development approach, not all groups work in a community development way. For example, groups do not 'fit' a community development approach if they are 'run' by the health visitor rather than facilitated and there is no opportunity for the sharing of knowledge, skills and authority. If the health visitor sets the agenda, organises the premises and the funding, then this group is not truly engaging in the empowerment process. Using this model, authority and power stay with the leader and the participants again become passive recipients of professional knowledge and skills. In contrast, in the self-help group the members hold the authority for the group and although a leader will emerge, the culture of the group and the task of the group determine that there is sharing of knowledge, mutual support and helping.

Self-help groups

Self-help groups are a common phenomenon of the community development movement. Here, people with similar difficulties meet and share feelings, thoughts and ideas and support each other emotionally and often practically. The key elements of self-help are: sharing a common experience, universality of sharing problems, reciprocity and mutual helping. Sometimes this collective experience leads to action and the group might lobby for new services or different ways of doing things, e.g. groups of parents campaigning for new services or funding for disabled children. It is the support element of self-help that makes it such a potent way of bringing about change, however. The experience of being involved with others whom they perceive as being like them helps members feel they are not alone with difficulties. Often their involvement moves them from a helpless role into a helping role and they use this validating experience of inclusion to build confidence and take action collectively with the support of others. This reduces isolation and the feelings of being overwhelmed by the task ahead as well as increasing opportunities for social interaction and developing new friendships.

Women's support groups

For many women the provision of a group is an opportunity just to get out of the house. The group is somewhere to go to have someone to talk to and to get help with difficulties. Research undertaken by Dalziel (1990) indicated that the women who go to such groups are usually young mothers with small children whose social condition often leaves them isolated and bored at home. The provision of a crèche and some time away from their children is one of the main reasons why women attend health groups.

The small group structure as a means of gaining social and emotional support appears to appeal to women more than men. This could be due to the focus in the group being on expressing feelings and sharing experiences, qualities often attributed to women. Men do get involved in supporting each other in groups but currently, it appears to be a mainly middle-class activity. Men's groups in the community do not appear to have the same appeal for working-class men although there is some evidence that this may be changing. The Danny Morrison Project in Drumchapel, Glasgow, is one example of how working-class men have begun to appreciate the value of groups and their cooperative and mutual support elements. Many women's groups run confidence-building, self-defence and complementary medicine classes, e.g. aromatherapy or reflexology. The sharing of experience and the sense of empowerment that participants gain seem to help disadvantaged groups build confidence and begin to articulate what they need for themselves.

Community profiling and needs assessment

One of the important benefits of community development is the ability to carry out needs assessments that reach into populations. It was discussed earlier how marginalised people often find it difficult to participate because of lack of confidence. Burton & Harrison (1997) believe that a community development approach to community profiling and needs assessment would help people be part of the process. Key features of a community development approach to needs assessment include:

- a process based on partnership and collaboration rather than a lone researcher;
- establishment and development of ongoing channels of communication rather than a snapshot of an area;
- commitment to give a voice to people not usually asked for views;
- a recognition and regard for qualitative as well as quantitative information;
- an acknowledgement of the process. Getting people together would then be seen as a major outcome.

The purpose of a community profile is usually to provide information from people's lived experience and the process often allows new local structures to develop as a framework evolves for allocation of tasks. The benefits can include that it:

- enables people to increase their knowledge about their community;
- encourages community initiative in finding people to do work;
- facilitates personal development;
- leads to acquisition of new skills;
- offers commissioning services a more meaningful evaluation of community need;
- provides a way of achieving a more democratic health service.

The information gathered is usually a combination of quantitative and qualitative data, including population statistics and demographic trends. The profile should also include information about the services and other resources in the area, such as churches, voluntary groups and statutory services, and the level of employment and occupational structure. Finally, community profiles include qualitative data regarding community members' views on the area, e.g. their perspectives on health priorities, service provision and what it is like to live in the area.

THE HEALTH VISITOR ROLE IN A COMMUNITY HEALTH PROJECT

One of the structures available to help health visitors work differently is the community health projects. In Scotland the first community health projects starting appearing in the 1980s. There are now an ever-increasing number in both the cities and rural areas.

Community health projects are usually located within areas of social and economic deprivation. They are funded from a variety of sources such as local authorities, health boards, health-care trusts, social work and charitable organisations like the Lottery or Carnegie Fund. The projects are staffed by workers from a variety of backgrounds, usually social work and community education but increasingly, as for health projects in Pilton in Edinburgh and Drumchapel in Glasgow, with a health visitor attachment.

Management of community health projects is often carried out by local people within a management committee structure and although the fine detail of their function might be different, health projects aim to offer support and practical help to enable communities to define and articulate their own health needs and then be part of addressing these needs. They also function to help the community achieve participatory competence. In their establishment and growth, they offer a manifest challenge to dominant systems like medicine, social work and education which are often perceived as marginalising and disempowering large sections of the community.

The author worked as a health visitor with a community development remit and set up community health projects. The case study below discusses that experience in order to illustrate the stages of the community development process and the role of the health visitor within the process. It also details what communities can achieve by working in this way.

Case study 8.1   Integration of health visitor caseload and community development work

From 1993 to 1997 the author held a post as a community development health visitor in Broomhouse, a poorly resourced area of Edinburgh. The initial remit was fairly wide and after some time, a caseload element was added to see if the approach could be integrated into a generic caseload. This case study explores the benefits and constraints of a community development process, including the issues around integration of community development and health visitor caseload work.
    The aims of the post were threefold:

1. to involve health visitors in community development initiatives;
2. to work with a community development approach with a defined community to address health issues;
3. to introduce a health perspective into the work of other professionals in the locality, e.g. community education, schools, police.

There are four distinct elements of the community development process: reflection, analysis, developing appropriate strategies and taking action. One element has an impact on the other which leads onto the next and so on in a continuous cycle. Several discrete stages of activities support the elements; some may overlap, some happen simultaneously and are difficult to separate, but they are all integral to the process.

Reflection: getting to know the community

This is the first stage and is often referred to as the 'hanging about' stage. For me, that involved visiting mother and toddler groups, women's groups, the local café and talking to people to find out who the key individuals in the community were. The purpose was to build up a picture of the community: the culture and values of the local people, what their needs were and where their interests and energy lay in addressing them.

Reflection: identifying structures and networks in the community

The next stage in the process (which overlapped to an extent with the first) was concerned with identifying the supports in the community. The area had few resources. There was a neighbourhood centre, two primary schools and two churches within Broomhouse and a community education centre just outside the area which was poorly used by Broomhouse residents. There was little voluntary activity or other opportunities for social contact. However, there was a group of people interested in being involved in addressing local health needs and they came together as the Broomhouse Health Strategy Group. With support, they eventually organised into a management committee, developed a constitution and created a set of aims and objectives for their work.

Analysis: working closely with local people to identify main concerns

One of the early pieces of work was a women's health day in the community education centre to encourage others to join the strategy group and begin the process of identifying need. This was successful with the membership, was enlarged and suggestions were made for a local women's group and support for mental health as future work.

Developing strategies: identifying with local people what needs to be done and establishing support

From this, the group decided to do a formal community needs assessment to discover other local health issues. Although the group acquired a grant and carried out research methods training for the members, the needs assessment was not completed due to resourcing difficulties (discussed in more detail below).

Developing strategies: clarifying opportunities for change

This stage was about identifying what needs to be done and how to go about doing it. Establishing the women's group was viewed as enlarging the opportunities for change and for further identification of need.

Taking action: with the community

Once the need is clarified and the strategy for change developed then the community is ready to take action. For example, the women's group started with support from local women and the community education centre.

Further reflection: coping with difficulties

The resourcing problems the group experienced with the needs assessment highlighted problems that are common to much of community health work.

Too much for too few

One of the difficulties the group faced at times was that in the process of taking action, there were too few people to do the work. For example, at the time of doing the survey there was a change in membership with four trained members leaving: one woman had a new baby and withdrew, two moved to another area and another one found employment. Getting volunteers involved in community work can be very difficult. An odd situation exists in community health projects where unemployed volunteers are encouraged to participate and are given training to help in this process. As a result, their confidence and skills are increased. This then makes them more able to get paid employment or involved in other community activities and community health projects rarely have sufficient resources to pay their valued volunteers. Volunteers leaving and moving on is often a criterion of success of a project but if they leave, the project is depleted and pressure is put on the ones remaining to attract more volunteers or to increase their own efforts. When this kind of work is more mainstream, then government-backed retraining money could help unemployed people remain in their community to undertake health-promoting work.

Too few resources for the task

As well as lack of people to carry out the planned needs assessment, there was no further money to carry out the tasks the initiative demanded, e.g. photocopying, support to analyse data and, as it was the wrong time of year for grants, a 'catch 22' situation prevailed. Projects like this which start from ground work need to be successful first and prove they can do the work before they will get properly funded. However, the lack of money to fund basics such as meetings, crèches and administrative support makes it more difficult for them to compete against core-funded projects in the search for money.

Naiveté about the complexity of needs assessment

The questionnaire developed from the volunteers training course was another constraining factor. The members piloted it with friends and family and concluded that the data resulting from this tool would be concerned with large public health issues like transport, crime and unemployment that we, as a small underfunded project, would not be able to address. The project members, all local people, were more interested at that time in people's private accounts of mental health, feelings and personal difficulties as opposed to socioeconomic needs, although we realised that they were not unconnected. The project was not resourced for addressing the wider issues being identified.

Further reflection: evaluating effectiveness of the action

Given all the problems, it was crucial for the project to review what had been achieved and decide on the positive and negative aspects of the experience. We agreed that community needs assessment is a very complex activity fraught with difficulties. It became obvious that the task was too big at that time for a part-time worker and a small group of volunteers with no administrative support and, consequently, the needs assessment was reluctantly abandoned. However, community development is about process outcomes as much as output indicators. The abandonment of the initiative meant there was no output but the next stage of reflecting on learning showed that the process outcomes were considerable.

Further reflection: planning new strategies for the future

From the reflection process, it was obvious that despite being unable to carry out the survey, the knowledge of the members and their understanding of health and research methods were considerably raised and, with this, their self-confidence. Training together also helped us become more of a team and we began to clarify and review our aims and objectives and to decide on what was manageable, given our limited resources.

Formal needs assessment had not been possible but instead the group decided to use their experience and local knowledge to create contact with the rest of the community. The methods they used to clarify the areas of need that interested them included:

- informal contact;
- holding training days on volunteering;
- small surveys;
- discussion groups;
- running a seminar on food;
- holding a conference on food issues.

Two of the main areas of need identified by the project were childcare and food work. Both are discussed here to demonstrate the process, activities and the issues involved.

Childcare

Through their experience of meeting together, the women's group identified that crèche provision and the delivery of crèche support locally were poor. When a crèche was needed the approach of the workers in the area was to employ local women with their sole qualifications being that they were mothers themselves and were available. They were untrained, there was no support for them to do the work, the pay was poor and consequently the service they offered was often less than satisfactory. The Health Strategy Group applied for money and invited the Playgroup Association to deliver training for local people wanting to work in crèches. The courses were so successful that other agencies asked to employ our crèche workers and soon the availability of training began to alter crèche policy in the area. Community Education eventually undertook to organise and fund the training and to compile a register of trained workers. The impact on the community of the crèche training was quite considerable, including:

- provision of employment for local women;
- offered new skills and knowledge;
- improved childcare in crèches;
- had some impact on the families of the crèche workers;
- changed local policy regarding employment and training of crèche workers.

Food work

The other important area of work identified by the Health Strategy Group addressed food issues locally. The diet in Broomhouse reflected the poor dietary status of other parts of Scotland and the group began to look at why this was so. It became apparent that the lack of local shops was a key feature. There was only one shop in the housing scheme which sold very little fruit or vegetables and what they did sell was of poor quality and highly priced. It was inevitable that, given the structural barriers of access, cost and quality and the prevailing food culture, people in the area bought little fruit and vegetables.

The strategy group approached the problem by holding a seminar and asking two other Edinburgh projects involved in food work to speak to them about setting up a fruit and vegetable co-op. The group decided to go ahead, secured some funding from Edinburgh Healthcare Trust and took over the lease of a shop for 6 months to test out the viability of the venture. It was a success from the very beginning, attracting over 100 members within the first year and recruiting new volunteers to the project.

The Broomhouse Food Project developed from this work as an independent project under the umbrella of the Health Strategy Group and became involved in other aspects of food work. The volunteers went into local schools and nurseries to introduce fruit into the tuck shops and persuaded the community café to introduce healthier choices. In alliance with Community Education and an Urban Aid Food Project (which some of them helped to start), they printed recipes, set up cooking skills classes and organised a Fun, Food and Football event for 80 local children with Hearts Football Club.

Impact on the community

Community development is a dynamic activity which uses feedback techniques to modify future activities and this makes it difficult to evaluate within conventional scientific research methodology. Beattie (1994) suggests four methods for evaluating the impact of community development as follows:

1. measuring outcomes;
2. monitoring process;
3. analysing client perspectives;
4. appraising institutional agendas.

The impact on the community from this piece of work was very considerable. Case studies of the volunteers and committee members were used in annual reports and funding applications to indicate shifts in client perspectives in relation to health. Informal data confirmed that their involvement in the project imperceptibly increased confidence and the ability to be further involved. Process descriptions of the project and its developments were also used to monitor progress. Outcome measurement and the shift in institutional agendas are used here to describe the impact the project had on new services and policy changes as follows.

New services established

- Counselling service
- Food project

- Fruit and vegetable co-op
- Women's project

Influence on local policy

- Community centres reduced sales of sweets and offered fruit to youth groups.
- Community café started offering wider variety of food and reduced the sale of fried food.
- Playgroups and nursery schools implemented a healthy eating policy.
- Local primary schools supplied fruit in tuck shops.
- Local GP fundholders provided core funding to sustain the project.

Increase in skills and knowledge locally

- Setting up of cooking classes
- Training of volunteers in food handling
- Training of volunteers in simple book-keeping skills
- Managing and running the co-op
- Managing meetings
- Team work training
- Listening and counselling skills
- Increase in knowledge about healthy eating
- Research methods training

Impact on poverty

- Reduced food costs
- Increased employment opportunities for crèche workers
- Establishment of the Credit Union

DISCUSSION: INTEGRATION OF CASELOAD AND COMMUNITY DEVELOPMENT WORK

It is clear from the examples of food work and childcare that nurses working alongside local people in this way can have a considerable impact on public health issues through influencing local policy to bring about structural changes. The important feature in the examples is the support of local people to define priorities and be part of the process of developing the services they require to achieve health gain. The process of community development, the involvement, the validation of knowledge and the collective action are important influences on individuals who participate and can lead to increased confidence and self-esteem, in itself health promoting. However, the structures within nursing that will support and encourage this kind of joint working with community members are not yet well established.

It was argued earlier that health visitors were well placed to take up the challenge of working differently to address inequalities in health but the question of how they will do it remains largely unanswered. Should the approach be integrated into the caseload or should there be community development specialists in small areas to support caseload workers? The experience of working both ways suggests that there are advantages and drawbacks with each approach.

There are benefits in having a health visitor with a caseload working in a community development way as opposed to a lone worker. One is the ready access to existing communities of interest, e.g. women with young children, older people or women in the antenatal period. Another is the general acceptance by other professionals of their role in community health. However, within the present structures and attached to group practices where the emphasis is on illness, individuals and a 'hands on' (usually dependent) relationship, the drawbacks are considerable.

Health visitor workloads are defined by their caseloads in two ways: structurally and emotionally. Having a caseload means spending time developing a relationship with individual families, being on call when they have a crisis, visiting them at home, seeing them in the clinic, being available to answer their questions, give advice and counsel and generally oversee the development of their under-5 children. This kind of work feeds our sense of being important and vital to others. It encourages us to know the answers and creates a dependence on patients for our knowledge and skills. The individualistic culture and medical model structures of the GP practice support the assumption that we, as nurses, can make things better. The statutory obligation to fulfil certain responsibilities for individual families also helps the concept and reality of the importance of the caseload work become very powerful. The small study carried out with health visitors trained in community development methods (Dalziel 1997) showed that given a choice between community development work or responding to caseload demands, the caseload won every time.

Community development work is not favoured because it is slow and for a while input will be largely invisible. It also involves nurses shedding the dependent, relatively distant professional relationship fostered by the caseload emphasis. Working with local people and using their knowledge demonstrates that they are the experts on themselves and although what we know is a valuable support to the work, it is not perceived to be more important than what they know. Given a choice, health visitors are drawn to fulfilling the caseload remit because it is clearer, more highly valued and, initially, emotionally more rewarding.

Working alone without a caseload and therefore without peers also has its drawbacks. It is lonely, often inadequately supported by management, poorly resourced and it is harder to make contacts. With a stated commitment to working with a community development approach throughout the health service and a willingness to adopt the changes this would entail, it should be possible to have several models of working with a community development approach. Health visitors could either have a split post or one designated post within the team. However, integration will only happen when the structures change and the community development way of working stops being marginal and becomes a mainstream method of addressing public and community health needs.

CONCLUSION

This chapter has shown that nurses can adopt community development methods in developing strategies to address public health issues. Health visitors in particular, with their history of public health nursing, have the necessary foundation on which to build new approaches to promoting health in communities.

To be truly effective in tackling deprivation and increasing health gain, nurses need to work within structures that support a more community-empowering approach to health inequalities. This means that their management must be knowledgeable about alternative approaches, can understand and encourage the philosophy of community development and is able to provide resources as well as supervision and personal support for the work.

Given the emphasis in community development on collectivity, equity, participation and empowerment, it is clear that nurses cannot be expected to work within primary care with this approach while primary care is dominated by a medical model of practice. The socioeconomic and environmental factors which are the key issues in deprivation will not be solved by medicine but by the redistribution of resources and by collaborative public health initiatives. The past hostility of the primary care structures to this way of working needs to be challenged if health visitors and other nurses are to stay within primary care and be able to fulfil community development and other public health remits.

Nurses can be involved in the achievement of the 'participatory competence' process (Kiefer 1983) referred to earlier, to enable local people to have a real voice in the policies affecting their health and well-being. The use of a community development approach to address public health issues demands that nurses work in a way that encourages partnership. A quote from Freeman (1997, p. 71) sums up this ethos: 'Working *on* a community may be regarded as manipulation, working *for* a community can be seen as a service, but working *with* a community will lead to real partnership'.

REFERENCES

Acheson D 1988 Public health in England. HMSO, London
Ashton J, Seymour H 1988 The new public health. Open University Press, Buckingham
Beattie A 1994 Health and well-being: a reader. Macmillan, London
Beigal D E 1984 Help seeking and receiving in urban ethnic neighbourhoods: strategies for empowerment. In: Rappaport J, Swift C, Hess R (eds) Studies in empowerment: steps towards understanding and action. Hawthorn Press, New York
Burton P, Harrison L 1997 Identifying local health needs. Policy Press, University of Bristol

Craig P 1998 A description of a public health role for health visitors. Unpublished MSc thesis, University of Glasgow

Dalziel Y 1990 The function of women's health groups in meeting health need in the community. Unpublished thesis, Edinburgh University

Dalziel Y 1997 Community development in primary care. Unpublished report. Edinburgh Healthcare NHS Trust, Edinburgh

Duffy S 1996 Partnerships in action. Health Education Board, Scotland

Freeman J 1997 The politics of women's liberation. King's Fund, London

Funnel R, Oldfield K, Speller V 1995 Towards healthier alliances. Health Education Authority, London

Hawe P 1994 Capturing the meaning of 'community' in community intervention evaluation: some contributions from community psychology. Health Promotion International 9(3): 199–209

Iscoe I 1974 Community psychology and the competent community. American Psychology 29: 607–613

Jones J 1990 Community development and health education: concepts and philosophy. Roots and Branches Papers from OU/HEA 1990 Winter School on Community Development and Health. Open University, Milton Keynes

Kiefer C H 1983 Citizen empowerment: a developmental perspective. Prevention in Human Services 3(23): 9–37

Lukes S 1978 Power: a radical view. Macmillan, London

Meleis A I 1992 Community participation and involvement: theoretical and empirical issues. Health Service Management Research 5(1): 5–16

OU/HEA 1990 Roots and branches. Papers from 1990 Winter School on Community Development and Health. Open University, Milton Keynes

Rappaport J, Swift C, Hess R (eds) 1984 Studies in empowerment: steps towards understanding and action. Hawthorn Press, New York

Sarason S B 1974 A psychological sense of community: prospects for a community psychology. Jossey Bass, San Francisco

Schiller P L, Levin J S 1983 Is self-care a social movement? Social Science and Medicine 17: 1343–1352

SNMAC 1995 Making it happen. Department of Health, London

Townsend P, Davidson N 1983 The Black report. Penguin

Watkins S J 1994 Public health 2020. British Medical Journal 309: 1147–1149

White J 1998 Health promotion and the public health role of health visitors: a report of research carried out in Bradford and Airedale. Bradford District Health Promotion Service, Shipley

WHO 1977 Alma-Ata: primary health care. World Health Organisation, UNICEF, Geneva

9

Communicable diseases

Joan Sneddon   Carol Fraser

INTRODUCTION

It is now over 40 years since the first infection control nurse (ICN) was appointed in the UK in 1959 in response to the pandemic staphylococcal infections of that decade (Worsley 1988). Further appointments slowly followed but it was not until the late 1980s and into the 1990s that ICNs were to be found in most acute hospitals. Traditionally infection control has been perceived as primarily being a matter of concern for hospitals. This view is now changing. The move in recent years to appoint ICNs to public health communicable diseases teams reflects the increasing awareness of infection as a major public health issue.

The belief that communicable diseases had been conquered by modern medicine was shattered by the advent of AIDS. Similarly, the emergence of methicillin-resistant *Staphylococcus aureus*, vancomycin-resistant enterococci and multidrug-resistant strains of *Mycobacterium tuberculosis* has shown that antibiotic 'wonder drugs' can no longer be relied on. As a result of these developments, in recent years, increasing emphasis has been placed on control measures to prevent transmission of infection in both hospitals and the wider community.

This chapter will explore the challenges facing public health departments in their efforts to protect the public from communicable diseases. The various components of communicable disease control will be discussed, with particular reference to the infection control nurse, including: the historical background and legislative context; the structure and function of public health department communicable diseases teams; and the relationship of public health legislation to the care of individual patients.

COMMUNICABLE DISEASES

Communicable diseases, sometimes referred to as 'infectious' or 'contagious' diseases, are defined as being 'caused by a living organism and transmitted from person to person or from animal or bird to man either directly or indirectly' (Donaldson & Donaldson 1993).

In order to produce disease an organism must gain entry to the body in sufficient quantity, commonly referred to as the 'infectious dose', to initiate the infection process (Monto et al 1991). To gain entry to the body, organisms use one or more transmission mechanisms (Fig. 9.1).

Although many professionals are involved in communicable disease control, organisation and management are the responsibility of public health departments. The function of public health departments in relation to communicable disease control is multifactorial, encompassing surveillance,

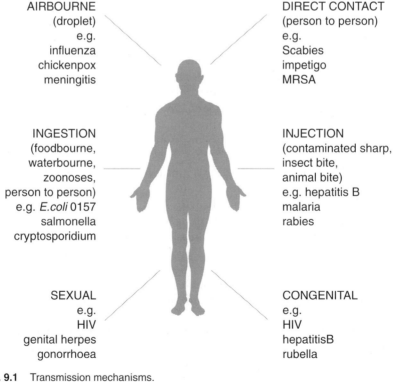

AIRBOURNE
(droplet)
e.g.
influenza
chickenpox
meningitis

DIRECT CONTACT
(person to person)
e.g.
Scabies
impetigo
MRSA

INGESTION
(foodbourne,
waterbourne,
zoonoses,
person to person)
e.g. *E.coli* 0157
salmonella
cryptosporidium

INJECTION
(contaminated sharp,
insect bite,
animal bite)
e.g. hepatitis B
malaria
rabies

SEXUAL
e.g.
HIV
genital herpes
gonorrhoea

CONGENITAL
e.g.
HIV
hepatitisB
rubella

Fig. 9.1 Transmission mechanisms.

outbreak management, infection control policy development and implementation and disease prevention initiatives.

Historical perspective

In early times illnesses were attributed to paranormal phenomena of good or evil, either the devil's work or a punishment from the gods. However, that certain diseases can be transmitted from one person to another has been recognised for centuries. Some believed that an object, a contagion, passed between people and caused disease, while others ascribed such illnesses to inhalation of toxic emanations or miasmas (Meers et al 1992).

In biblical times lepers were isolated to prevent transmission of infection and in the 14th century, at the time of the bubonic plague, doctors wore protective clothing and respirators stuffed with herbs to shield themselves. Not until true microbiology developed in the late 19th century was the existence of bacteria and viruses and their role in infectious diseases clarified (Caddow 1989).

Long before micro-organisms were identified, public health measures to control the spread of infection were being employed; the idea is not new. In Babylonia, well before the time of Christ, it was the practice to burn the clothing of infectious disease cases and bury the dead well away from where people lived. The importance of protecting the water supply from contamination was also recognised and the later contribution of the Romans to public health with the introduction of fresh water delivery and sewerage systems is well documented.

In 1796 Edward Jenner experimented with extracting pus from a cowpox lesion on the hand of a dairymaid with which he successfully inoculated James Phipps, thus protecting him from smallpox (Donaldson & Donaldson 1993). This first vaccine was the origin of the science of artificially created acquired immunity. It was a great success, taking less than 200 years to eradicate the disease, with the world being declared smallpox free in 1979 (DoH et al 1996a).

Also in the 18th century, John Pringle, a British Army physician, suggested that diseases might be caused by dirt and introduced the concept of hygiene into army hospitals. Then later, in 1847, Ignas Semmelweiss demonstrated the importance of handwashing to prevent the transmission of infection (Meers et al 1992).

The basic principles of public health measures to control the transmission of communicable diseases have therefore evolved over a long period.

ORGANISATIONAL FRAMEWORK FOR COMMUNICABLE DISEASE CONTROL

Communicable disease control was one of the earliest functions of public health and remains a major component to this day, with health boards (health authorities in England and Wales) and local authorities sharing this statutory responsibility (NHS (Scotland) Act 1978). Prior to 1974, communicable disease control was the responsibility of the public health departments of each local authority.

In 1974 there was a reorganisation of the NHS and local government. At this time many former local government functions were transferred to the NHS, one of which was the medical component of communicable disease control. The main changes were the abolition of the post of medical officer of health of the local authorities (LA) and the transfer of the duties of the post to the chief administrative medical officer (CAMO) of the health board acting as the designated medical officer to the LA. The consultant in public health medicine (CPHM) with a main interest in communicable diseases and environmental health, known as the consultant in communicable disease control (CCDC) in England and Wales, in practice undertakes the day-to-day aspects of communicable disease control and also acts as the designated medical officer (proper officer in England and Wales) of the local authority.

Current legislative framework

In Scotland the Infectious Diseases (Notification) Act 1889 and the Public Health (Scotland) Act 1897, in addition to subsequent updates and amendments, form the legal basis for control of communicable diseases. Similar legislation applies in other parts of the United Kingdom. The NHS (Scotland) Acts of 1972 and 1978 transferred the authority of the medical officer of health to the CAMO. The requirement for the notification of specified infectious diseases and also the legal powers for measures to control the spread of disease, e.g. the exclusion of infected persons from work or school and the hospitalisation of infected persons for treatment, are contained within these Acts.

Health board public health departments (PHDs), in conjunction with LA environmental health departments, have legal responsibility for the control of communicable diseases among the entire population within their geographical area, including NHS staff and patients.

The role of the health board department of public health

To fulfil public health responsibilities in relation to communicable disease control, PHDs must ensure that arrangements are in place for surveillance, investigation, prevention and control of communicable diseases (SODH 1996).

Surveillance, the methodical accumulation of data related to cases or carriers of infectious diseases, enables the detection of further cases, the identification of outbreaks or epidemics and the initiation of appropriate control measures (Donaldson & Donaldson 1993). Good surveillance is reliant on the rapid identification of the specific organism responsible for an illness (SODHAGI 1996).

People with symptoms suggestive of a communicable illness must be thoroughly investigated to ascertain the cause. Only in this way is it possible to initiate effective treatment of cases and, if indicated, trace other potential cases and contacts. The nature of the individual disease dictates the need for further investigations, which are undertaken by the PHD in collaboration with the local authority and other relevant agencies, e.g. the water authorities, the state veterinary service and the Health and Safety Executive.

As a consequence of investigations the CPHM may recommend that specific control measures are enforced to prevent further spread or recurrence of infection (SODHAGI 1996). These may necessitate the immediate closure of premises, the exclusion of food handlers from work or advice on hygiene practices.

Health boards also have an important role in promoting health. Many communicable diseases can be prevented and the provision of advice and education on measures which can interrupt the infection chain is a major component of the work of PHDs, both at a strategic level and on an ad hoc basis. Prevention of communicable diseases particularly related to childhood illnesses has been hugely influenced by immunisation programmes coordinated by PHDs.

The communicable diseases team

In Scotland, PHD communicable diseases teams usually have at least one consultant in public health medicine (CCDC in England and Wales). It is recognised, however, that PHDs can benefit from input from a wider variety of professionals (NHSME 1996, SE 1996) and many have an ICN within their communicable diseases team. ICNs have the specialist knowledge required for this essential part of the health board responsibility, bringing skills from a different background to complement those of their medical colleagues.

Role of the ICN working within a PHD

The role of the ICN is similar in many ways to that of the CPHM responsible for the control of communicable diseases. However, while participating in most aspects of communicable disease control, their work is generally nearer to the 'coalface', reflecting the more practical aspects of their knowledge and experience of hands-on infection control. Key functions include the development of links with the primary, secondary and tertiary care sectors and the provision of advice, support and education to health and social care professionals, voluntary organisations, schools, nurseries and the general public regarding prevention, treatment and control of infection (see case studies below)

Infection control committees

Health boards have a responsibility to ensure that control of infection policies and procedures are in place to deal with routine infection problems and outbreaks of infection. Health board infection control advisory committees (HBICAC) can assist them to fulfil this function (SODHAGI 1998, DoH 1995). Committee membership usually includes the CPHM responsible for communicable disease control as chairperson, the public health infection control nurse (PHICN) and representatives of local trust infection control teams, microbiologists, hospital clinicians, general practice, environmental health and occupational health departments. HBICACs are important sources of expert advice, helping to maintain a coordinated approach to control of infection by defining standards, recommending policies, providing a forum for liaison between health boards and NHS trusts and monitoring local infection control services. NHS trusts have their own local control of infection committees who monitor the incidence of infection within their area and ensure the maintenance of good infection control practice. Committee membership is drawn from relevant disciplines within trusts and includes, as a representative of the health board, the CPHM and in some areas the PHICN. Trust infection control teams, which usually consist of a consultant microbiologist and at least one ICN, are responsible for the routine day-to-day surveillance and management of infection within the trust, liaising with the PHD where appropriate (SODHAGI 1998, DoH 1995).

NOTIFICATION AND SURVEILLANCE OF COMMUNICABLE DISEASES

In the Western world, communicable diseases are no longer the mass killers of previous centuries. Nevertheless, deaths still occur and communicable diseases are an important cause of morbidity and premature mortality. Emerging new infections and reemerging old infections cause both professional and public concern and much media attention.

The statutory notification of certain specified infectious diseases (Fig. 9.2), is the legal responsibility of the attending medical practitioner. This system, which has been in place for the past 100 years, requires doctors to complete notification forms and submit them to the health board. It is the main source of information on the occurrence of infectious diseases but has been augmented more recently by regular reports supplied directly from microbiology laboratories. Laboratory data can be particularly helpful in quickly identifying outbreaks or clusters of infection. Whilst written notification is required by law, early notification by telephone is encouraged for those infections which require urgent investigation and control measures, e.g. meningococcal meningitis and some gastrointestinal pathogens. The information obtained is used on a daily basis by PHDs to initiate follow-up investigations and the prompt introduction of appropriate control measures.

Anthrax	Poliomyelitis
Bacillary dysentry	Puerperal fever
Chickenpox	Rabies
Cholera	Relapsing fever
Diphtheria	Rubella
Erysipelas	Scarlet fever
Food poisoning	Smallpox
Legionellosis	Tetanus
Leptospirosis	Toxoplasmosis
Lyme disease	Tuberculosis:
Malaria	respiratory
Measles	non-respiratory
Membranous croup	Tyhoid fever
Meningococcal infection	Typhus fever
Mumps	Viral haemorrhagic fevers
Paratyhoid fever	Viral hepatitis
Plague	Whooping cough

Fig. 9.2   Notifiable diseases in Scotland (source: SODHAGI 1996).

The routine collection, close scrutiny and dissemination of information on the occurrence of communicable diseases enables clusters of infection to be identified and local disease trends to be monitored which facilitates emergency and strategic planning of communicable disease control measures. In Scotland, local information is forwarded to the Scottish Centre for Infection and Environmental Health (SCIEH) for inclusion in national data. National surveillance data is published by the SCIEH regularly in their 'Weekly Report', therefore information on both local and national trends is quickly available to PHDs. In addition, most PHDs disseminate local epidemiological information to health professionals in their own area in regular newsletters. Similar mechanisms exist in other parts of the UK.

OUTBREAK MANAGEMENT

Outbreaks of infection regularly occur and commonly they are foodborne. Foodborne diseases are often referred to as 'food poisoning', a general term applied to any disease where the cause is known or thought to be infectious or toxic and resulting from consumption of contaminated water or food (SODHAGI 1996). The responsibility for investigating foodborne diseases rests jointly with the PHD of health boards and environmental health departments of local authorities. On receipt of a notification of food poisoning, the PHD arranges for the person to be interviewed, usually by an environmental health officer (EHO). A detailed account of the illness and a food history is obtained. From the information collected, it may be possible to identify links with other cases and form a working hypothesis on the possible cause.

While persons suffering from gastrointestinal infections continue to have diarrhoea there is an increased risk of spread to others either directly or via food, particularly if hygiene standards are poor. For this reason cases are asked to stay off work or school until they have been clinically well for 48 hours and the EHO will give advice on personal and food hygiene. Some persons fall into groups considered to be at special risk of spreading infection (SODHAGI 1996) and can be excluded from school or work until declared clear of the infecting organism. This statutory power is used less now than in the past as it is recognised that for the majority of gastrointestinal infections the risk of transmission is negligible when diarrhoea has ceased, the person is passing formed stools and hand hygiene is good.

PHDs have formal plans based on national guidance (SODHAGI 1996) to deal with outbreaks of infection. Early recognition of outbreaks is essential to enable prompt action to be initiated. Appropriate people must be informed quickly and an outbreak control team established. Outbreaks must be investigated thoroughly, promptly and systematically. Only in this way can sources of infection and transmission mechanisms be identified and appropriate measures to prevent spread be initiated.

Case study 9.1   *Escherichia coli* O157

In 1996 a major outbreak of *Escherichia coli* O157 infection occurred in central Scotland. The outbreak was identified when on Friday 22 November the PHD of Lanarkshire Health Board became aware of 10 possible and five provisionally positive cases of *E. coli* O157. All but one of the cases came from the area around Wishaw, a town in Lanarkshire with a population of approximately 30 000. Eight of the cases were in hospital and seven in the community. Investigations were initiated immediately with nine people being interviewed by 1700 hours that evening. All but one of those interviewed had either eaten cold meat products originating from a local butcher or steak pie supplied by the same butcher served at a church lunch on 17 November 1996. This indication of a probable common source prompted action that evening to stop distribution of the foods implicated. An extensive supply chain to other food outlets throughout central Scotland was later revealed through the further investigations of the LA.

An outbreak control team (OCT) was established in line with national guidance (SODH 1996) and met on a daily basis to investigate the outbreak. The investigation was split into four distinct elements, as shown in Figure 9.3

After identification of the outbreak the number of suspected cases rapidly grew. The outbreak was centred in Lanarkshire where 380 confirmed and suspected cases occurred. The total for the entire central Scotland outbreak was 502 cases, mainly in Lanarkshire and The Forth Valley. Of those infected, 21 died, all of whom were over 65 years of age. The epidemic curve (Fig. 9.4) of the dates of onset of symptoms in the cases for whom this information was known demonstrated a pattern in line with an ongoing point source outbreak.

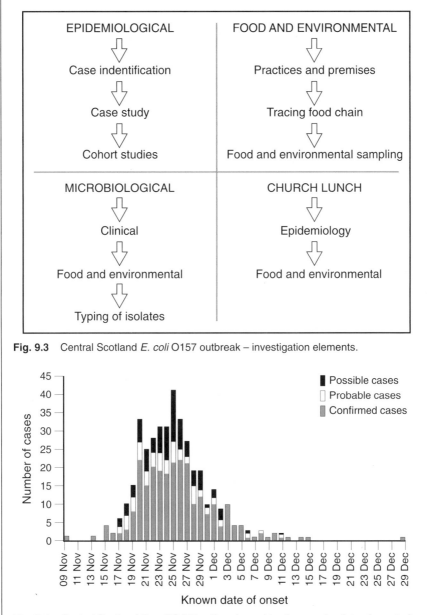

Fig. 9.3 Central Scotland *E. coli* O157 outbreak – investigation elements.

Fig. 9.4 Central Scotland *E. coli* O157 outbreak – epidemic curve by date of onset of diarrhoea.

The *E. coli* O157 isolated from the stool samples of cases was typed as phage type 2, VT1 negative, VT2 positive. *E. coli* O157 of the same phage type was also isolated from both environmental and food samples taken from the premises of the butcher. The DNA profile of isolates from the human cases and food and environmental samples were indistinguishable.

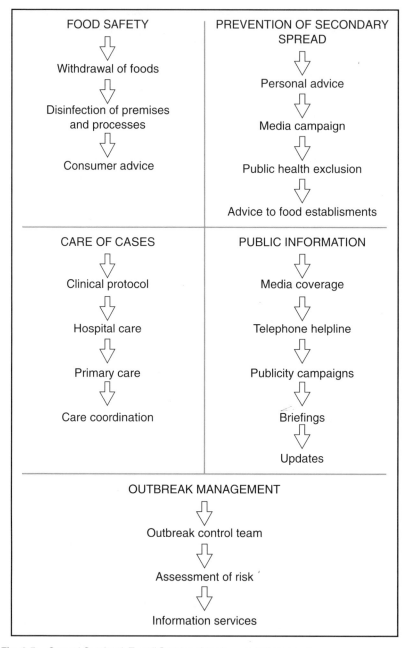

Fig. 9.5 Central Scotland *E. coli* O157 outbreak – control measures.

In addition to the ongoing investigation, the OCT were responsible for ensuring that appropriate arrangements were in place to care for those infected and to control the outbreak. Comprehensive control measures were instituted, as shown in Figure 9.5.

The outbreak caused much public anxiety, particularly amongst the population of Wishaw. A community outbreak clinic was established in Wishaw Health Centre to support the GPs and a total of 924 people attended this over a 4-week period with many more attending other GPs throughout Lanarkshire. In all, during the outbreak, information was accumulated on 2662 individuals, 14 507 clinical specimens were collected and 1411 food and 206 environmental samples taken.

Media interest was intense and to help allay public concern, a telephone helpline was established with 1182 calls being received. Other measures included daily press releases, interviews, public information leaflet distribution and advertisements in local and national press.

ICNs were involved in all aspects of the management and control of the outbreak. The PHICN served as a regular member of the OCT, maintained a liaison function with all the agencies involved in the outbreak, participated in the collection, coordination and analysis of data, helped in the preparation of public information leaflets and briefing guidance to professionals and provided advice to nursing and residential homes.

The Wishaw Outbreak Clinic was managed and run by the ICNs from the local community NHS trust. Here people were monitored for signs and symptoms of *E. coli* O157 infection and were given advice on hand and food hygiene and other measures to prevent secondary spread. The ICNs also liaised with the acute hospital trusts on a regular basis about cases admitted to and discharged from hospital care.

Cases who required hospital care were nursed in two local acute hospitals. The large numbers of patients admitted necessitated the allocation of additional beds for isolation nursing. Many staff unfamiliar with and anxious about caring for patients requiring isolation nursing were required to care for cases. A major role of the hospital ICNs at this time was to provide support, training and advice. The ICNs interviewed and took detailed food histories from cases, coordinated supplies, kept track of admissions and discharges and liaised with Lanarkshire Health Board and the community clinic in Wishaw.

The outbreak demonstrated the importance of teamwork. Close liaison and cooperation between PHDs, local authorities and the primary and secondary health-care sectors was vital and without it the situation would have been impossible to manage and control effectively. This was acknowledged in the report of the Pennington Group (1997) which was set up by the government to report on the outbreak and the circumstances leading up to it, as well as the implications for food safety and the lessons to be learned.

CONTROL OF INFECTION POLICIES, PROCEDURES AND GUIDELINES

In order to fulfill their public health responsibilities, health boards/ authorities need to have policies, procedures and guidelines covering all aspects of communicable disease control within their area. The development of such guidance is a function of health board infection control advisory committees and is coordinated by the PHDs.

National expert bodies regularly review surveillance and epidemiological data, research findings, technological advances, therapeutic interventions and legislative changes and produce guidance on best practice in the management, treatment and control of various specific infectious diseases and infection control in general. Local guidance is developed by task-specific working groups with membership drawn from the professional expertise represented on health board infection control advisory committees.

When preparing health board guidance, working groups consider national guidance documents along with local epidemiology, organisational structures, strategic planning and clinical expertise. Policies, procedures and guidelines prepared at health board level may require adaptation within specific health-care settings to reflect differing operational arrangements.

Control of infection in hospitals and community trusts

Health boards have to 'ensure adequate infection control arrangements within hospitals' and to secure the 'support of the hospital in infection control in the community' (DoH 1995). In the mid-1990s, in the purchaser–provider era, these objectives were achieved through inclusion of specific infection control quality standards in contracts. The demise of the internal market and health board contracts with service providers (SODH 1997) in no way diminishes the importance of such standards or the responsibility of health boards to monitor the quality of provision of health care delivered by trusts.

Whilst the standards set by individual health boards will vary to reflect the specific priorities for the health of their population, core elements should be common to all and should be agreed with trusts.

Trusts need to have effective organisational structures, with clear lines of accountability for infection control services to facilitate the routine surveillance, investigation, control and prevention of infection. There should be a requirement for trusts to fulfil their routine responsibilities under public health legislation and also to notify the PHD of any significant public health incident or outbreak of infection. They must also develop emergency plans detailing their response in the event of outbreaks of communicable disease either within their own service or in the wider community. Mechanisms should be in place to develop and adjust systems as necessary, to adopt changes to local health board and Department of Health policies, procedures, best practice guidelines and legislative requirements. This includes the maintenance of staff awareness about infection control by ongoing education and training progammes and the demonstration of good practice by ongoing active audit programmes. Some health boards require specific infection rate data, commonly for surgical procedures (Hospital Infection Working Group 1995).

PHDs monitor the infection control activities of trusts in a variety of ways. Through membership of trust infection control committees, the CPHM and/or the PHICN can contribute to the development and monitoring of hospital policies and have cognisance of the issues being brought to the committee for discussion, including hospital-acquired infection data. Additionally, involvement in the management of incidents and outbreaks of infection within trusts gives first-hand knowledge of the functioning of the infection control services. Trusts are usually required to submit an annual report on their infection control activities for the preceding year and their planned programme for the forthcoming year. This should include proposed activity related to surveillance of infected patients, audit of standards and education and training of hospital staff (SODHAGI 1998, SODH 1999). Monitoring information is reviewed by the PHD and the health board infection control advisory committee and is taken into consideration when advice is provided to the health board on infection control issues.

Advisory role

Over the last decade there has been a shift of service provision towards the primary care setting. This has occurred as a result of the NHS reforms based on the *Promoting better health* (1987), *Working for patients* (1989) and *Caring for people* (1989) White Papers and the NHS and Community Care Act 1990. Patients now spend less time in hospital. Many susceptible patients are being managed in the primary care setting, including having invasive diagnostic and therapeutic procedures carried out. The potential for infection and crossinfection is substantial. PHDs provide control of infection advice in all community settings to health and social care staff as well as to the general public.

Primary care

Infection control in the primary care settings has in the past attracted less attention than in hospitals although some studies have identified poor infection control practice (Morgan et al 1990, Sneddon et al 1997). PHDs have a responsibility to ensure the quality of infection control practice in the primary care setting as they do throughout the health board area. ICNs, with their specialist knowledge, practical experience and access to relevant guidelines and policies, are well equipped to provide advice and guidance. They can provide information, advice and training relevant to specific communicable disease and to infection control in general. Of particular importance are decontamination and sterilisation procedures for surgical instruments in order to protect the public from the risk of transmission of infections, including bloodborne viruses such as HIV, hepatitis B and C.

As employers, general medical and dental practitioners have a statutory responsibility under the terms of the Health and Safety at Work Act 1974 to maintain a safe environment. They should have comprehensive, relevant infection control policies which are 'specific to the practice, its personnel and equipment' (Cooke 1993); only in this way can consistency be ensured (Sneddon et al 1997). The ICN is a useful resource for practices developing policies and some PHDs have produced, distributed and regularly review core guidance on which such practice policies can be based.

Despite the increase in minor surgery carried out in general medical practice, no national quality standards for these procedures in this setting exist. When procedures move from the secondary to the primary care setting the same clinical standards should apply and health boards have a responsibility to ensure that they do (NHSME 1996). Some PHDs have therefore developed their own local standards agreed with general practitioners and are working towards their implementation.

Long-term residential care

Both the ageing population and the advent of community care have resulted in an increase in the number of residential and nursing homes. In such settings where there are many elderly frail people, some of whom have invasive devices such as urinary catheters in situ, there is a risk of the spread of infection. Whilst such establishments endeavour to create as homely an environment as possible, it is important that a good standard of infection control practice is maintained as a matter of routine. All staff, both professional and untrained, have a role to play in control of infection and must have access to and be familiar with infection control policies relevant to their duties. Training and regular updating are essential. Some PHICNs have introduced infection control link nurse systems which enable them to train and regularly update a designated nurse in each home who can then act as a resource and cascade information on control of infection issues to other staff.

National guidance on infection control in nursing and residential homes has been published by the Department of Health (PHMEG 1996) and many PHDs have also produced and distributed local guidance on topics such as universal precautions, personal hygiene, cleaning and disinfection, laundry procedures, clinical waste, management of invasive devices and food hygiene.

An evolving issue

Many microorganisms which are responsible for hospital-acquired infection have often been dismissed when they occur in the community. This attitude has begun to change mainly as a result of the shift of emphasis in health-care delivery from the secondary to the primary care setting. Patients in more acute stages of illness are being cared for in nursing or residential homes or in their own home and this, along with the increase in invasive treatments and procedures performed, has resulted in microorganisms once primarily associated with hospital-acquired infection becoming increasingly significant in the community setting.

One such microorganism which is now having a major impact in the community is methicillin-resistant *Staphylococcus aureus* (MRSA). MRSA was first identified shortly after the introduction of the antibiotic methicillin as a treatment for *Staphylococcus aureus* infections (Rontree & Beard 1968) in the early 1960s. Incidence remained generally low and mainly hospital associated throughout the 1970s and 1980s although outbreaks of MRSA within long-term care establishments were reported (Strausbaugh et al 1993).

Case study 9.2 MRSA

A 76-year-old lady, Mrs C, was identified as having MRSA during a hospital admission following a stroke. The initial positive specimen was a wound swab from a chronic leg ulcer which had exhibited signs of infection. A follow-up MRSA screen also identified nose and throat carriage.

Mrs C was nursed in isolation in a single room, according to hospital policy, and treatment for her MRSA infection was instituted. The treatment successfully resolved the wound infection but despite two further attempts to clear the nasal and throat carriage, these sites remained positive. As there were no clinical signs of infection and she was generally improving, no further treatment for the MRSA was indicated.

Steady progress was maintained but because of nursing and general needs as a result of her stroke, it was agreed that Mrs C required long-term nursing care which would be more appropriately delivered in a nursing home setting. Local authority social services are responsible for the coordination of care in the community and a social worker liaised with Mrs C and her family to identify a suitable nursing home.

A nursing home was approached to assess the suitability of their facilities for Mrs C's care requirements. This necessitated the nursing home matron meeting Mrs C and her family to carry out an assessment and at this time she was informed of the MRSA status. In principle, the matron agreed to Mrs C's admission to the home but the diagnosis caused concern. The nursing home had no previous experience of MRSA and on observing the management in hospital, the matron was unsure how her staff would react, especially in the light of recent sensationalised media reporting of the subject.

In order to alleviate possible concerns, the matron held a staff meeting to discuss MRSA management. The meeting highlighted many issues, especially the fear that other residents and also the staff themselves would 'catch' MRSA. As a result, admission to the home was postponed to allow time to seek advice, allay anxieties and ensure Mrs C's care needs could be met.

The matron contacted the PHD, the initial enquiry being received by the CPHM. The call was referred on to the PHICN, who had the specialist knowledge of the recommended infection control standards for nursing homes.

The PHICN initially discussed MRSA in general and advised on management, highlighting the reasons why care guidelines for hospitals vary from those recommended for the nursing home setting. The discussion was followed up by written information for staff and an offer to visit and discuss the issues with them was extended.

The delay in transfer to the nursing home upset Mrs C and her family and the help of the hospital ICN was enlisted to explain the situation and reassure them that any problems would soon be resolved.

Three days after the telephone call between the matron and PHD, the matron requested a visit from the PHICN to speak to staff who continued to have concerns. The visit took place 4 days later when the PHICN addressed the concerns raised by staff which revolved around mode of spread, pathogenicity, management of laundry, use of protective clothing, domestic hygiene, staff health and the importance of maintaining basic hygiene standards and, in particular, hand hygiene. The discussion with the PHICN enabled staff to air their concerns and allowed each issue to be directly addressed. The anxieties of staff were allayed and they were reassured by the support provided.

Two days later the matron contacted the social worker responsible for coordinating Mrs C's care and informed her the home was happy for the admission to go ahead, which it did the following week. Follow-up enquiries by the PHICN revealed that Mrs C had settled well into the home and staff had encountered no problems with her care.

During the 1990s the incidence of MRSA in hospitals noticeably increased and with it came a similar increase in the community. This increase highlighted the need for the appropriate management of MRSA in the community to be clarified. As a result, in 1995, the first guidelines for the control of

MRSA in community settings were published in a report of a combined Working Party of the British Society for Antimicrobial Chemotherapy and the Hospital Infection Society (Duckworth & Heathcock 1995).

As with other infection control issues, PHDs have a responsibility to disseminate information and provide practical guidance on management of MRSA to multidisciplinary community care teams, e.g. staff of day centres and nursing and residential homes, community care teams and domiciliary care services and the general public. In many health boards and health authorities, the role of ensuring that appropriate care is delivered and levels of hygienic practice are maintained is undertaken by the PHICN.

PREVENTION OF COMMUNICABLE DISEASES

Contact tracing

The action taken by PHDs on notification of infectious diseases is influenced by the nature of the infection, its communicability and perceived risks to others. For certain specific infectious diseases, contact tracing is a routine element in the management of the case.

Contact tracing is undertaken when an infectious disease poses a risk to others. Usually this applies to the household and very close associates of the case who may also have been exposed to the infection, as for example in tuberculosis or meningococcal disease. Tracing may be extended to a wider group if there are special considerations, e.g. increased susceptibility of a contact or the occurrence of a clustering of cases. The period of surveillance is dependent on the disease, e.g. contacts of patients with smear-positive tuberculosis should be followed up for at least 1 year (DoH et al 1996b). Contacts may require monitoring for signs of infection, chemoprophylaxis or immunisation.

It is usual for PHDs to formulate policy guidance on contact tracing within their area. Such guidance identifies the person(s) who will carry out the procedures and defines their roles and responsibilities. CPHMs often request the PHICN to undertake contact tracing for meningococcal disease. However, because of the volume of work required for tuberculosis, a full-time designated tuberculosis liaison nurse, usually a health visitor, is commonly contracted to undertake this role.

Often when cases requiring contact tracing occur, there is widespread public anxiety fuelled by rumour and media reporting. Part of the PHD's response to such situations is to offer reassurance to the general public by the provision of information about the particular infection and the degree of risk to the wider community. For example, when a case of meningococcal disease has occurred, it is common practice to contact the school or nursery involved and arrange for letters and information leaflets to be distributed to the parents of the other children.

Immunisation

Immunisation has played a key role in the decline of infectious diseases over the past 100 years. Many vaccines have been developed using Jenner's principles and are now used to vaccinate (immunise) against a variety of infectious diseases.

Vaccination works by stimulating the immune system to produce antibodies against specific diseases, resulting in active immunity to that disease. The immunity is generally long-lasting but for some diseases booster doses are required.

One objective of the 'Alma-Ata declaration' (WHO 1978), which was agreed by the world's nations, was to immunise the population of the world against the majority of infectious diseases. To date, this objective has not been achieved, primarily due to the restricted resources available to public health to implement and maintain immunisation programmes. This, together with an increase in world travel and microorganisms developing resistance to antibiotics, has contributed to the re-emergence of old infectious diseases, for example tuberculosis.

The aim of immunisation is twofold: to protect an individual against serious or life-threatening disease and to protect the community as a whole, commonly referred to as herd immunity. The success of immunisation programmes is influenced by other factors such as continued surveillance, a key PHD function, and the existence of environmental and animal reservoirs. To prioritise immunisation programmes it is essential to understand the epidemiology of infectious diseases. For example, in 1992, surveillance identified changes in the age distribution of measles. This resulted in the initiation of a mass measles-rubella immunisation programme, undertaken in 1994, to minimise the risk of a measles epidemic. The programme proved to be successful with a marked rapid decrease in cases being reported (DoH et al 1996a).

As a component of the NHS general medical services to the population, the Department of Health provide a childhood immunisation programme (DoH et al 1996a). PHDs are responsible for the coordination and monitoring of this programme which is delivered by general practitioners and child and school health services. They also provide an advisory service to professionals on any issues relating to immunisation.

Travel immunisation

World travel is becoming increasingly popular and people are being exposed to infectious diseases which are uncommon in the UK. The speed of travel enables people to visit a variety of countries in a short period of time. They can therefore be exposed to infection in one country and, because of the incubation period, return to the UK before developing symptoms.

Travellers must be aware of the risks from infection when travelling abroad. However, many factors contribute to the risk and must be taken into account when giving advice, e.g. specific infections which may be encountered, the duration of stay, planned activities, mode of travel, type of accommodation, their own general health and need for emergency first aid supplies (DoH et al 1995).

Practical advice on preventive measures is of equal or greater importance than the reliance on vaccination or prophylactic medication. For example, only about 5% of travel-related illness is preventable by vaccination (Richards & Whitfield 1995).

PHDs often receive enquiries regarding travel health and are able to offer general advice. They may also issue the Department of Health booklet which gives health advice for travellers anywhere in the world and is updated on an annual basis (DoH 1997). Travel medicine is, however, a rapidly changing field and for specific guidance callers are usually referred on for expert advice to specially designated travel clinics run by, for example, specialist infectious diseases units.

Health promotion

Health promotion is a concept which developed with the modern public health movement with its key aim of improving health and addressing problems of diseases and their consequences. This emerged in 1974 when the Canadian government released the report of Marc Lalonde which proposed that the health of the public could be improved by focusing on prevention rather than cure (Lalonde 1974).

As a result of Lalonde's report, in 1976, the Department of Health and Social Security published the consultative document *'Prevention and health: everybody's business'* which influenced the direction of PHDs' health promotion activities thereafter. The currently favoured model of health promotion revolves around the interlinked themes of education, prevention and protection (Tannahill 1985).

Health education is about communication, providing health-related information and learning opportunities with the intention to produce 'some relatively permanent changes in understanding or ways of thinking' (Tones 1986) in order to influence individuals to change beliefs or attitudes about health and to adopt healthier lifestyles.

Prevention is another major component of which there are three levels.

1. *Primary prevention*, which aims to prevent disease occurring by changing the behaviour or the status of the host, for example by immunisation or the enforcement of food hygiene principles. It has been responsible for many successes in reducing the incidence of specific infectious diseases. The reduction in reported cases of measles as a result

of the 1994 measles, mumps and rubella immunisation programme is one such example, as is the dramatic reduction in the incidence of cases of *Haemophilus influenzae* meningitis following the introduction of Hib vaccine in 1992 (DoH et al 1996a).

2. *Secondary prevention* aims to halt the progression of disease and relies for its success on early detection and prompt intervention, e.g. screening of immigrants for tuberculosis.

3. *Tertiary prevention*, which aims to minimise complications resulting from established disease, improving quality of life but not necessarily curing the disease, as is the case in the follow-up of HIV, hepatitis B and C cases.

Health protection measures are designed to prevent disease by ensuring recommended practice is in place and maintained. Measures include legal controls, regulations, policies or voluntary codes of practice, e.g. the Health and Safety at Work Act 1974 and the Food Safety Act 1994.

The three elements of health promotion can and do overlap and require a community-wide approach which involves the multidisciplinary collaboration of both statutory and voluntary organisations if it is to be effective. PHDs have a key role to play in the coordination of activities which promote health and prevent disease and in maintaining surveillance programmes which can identify 'problems' and enable preventive control measures to be instituted.

Case study 9.3   HIV and hepatitis

Health promotion to a larger or lesser degree has a role to play in the management of most communicable diseases and this particularly applies to the bloodborne viruses, e.g. HIV and hepatitis B and C.

HIV/AIDS is one of the most serious threats to the public health, both nationally and internationally, which has emerged in recent years. The first case of AIDS was diagnosed in 1981 although the human immunodeficiency virus was not isolated until 1983 (SHAIR Group 1995). Current evidence suggests that most people with HIV infection will eventually go on to develop AIDS, about half doing so within 10 years of contracting the infection. It is estimated that a high proportion of cases will die.

The virus is transmitted in three ways:

1. by unprotected penetrative sexual intercourse with an infected person (between men or between men and women);
2. through infected blood, which in the UK is usually as a result of intravenous drug users sharing injecting equipment but can also occur from accidental exposure as a result of a contaminated 'sharps' injury;
3. from an infected mother to her baby either before or during birth or through breast feeding.

Sustained changes in sexual or drug-using behaviour, i.e. safer sexual practices and the use of clean injecting equipment and its safe disposal, are necessary if transmission is to be prevented.

Policy related to the prevention of HIV transmission in Scotland was the subject of a Ministerial Task Force Report (SOHHD 1992) which made comprehensive recommendations. These were later reinforced by the Ministerial Task Force on Drugs (SOHHD 1994). The significant growing problem of drug misuse was acknowledged in both reports, as was the need to take a broad approach to HIV prevention to include harm reduction initiatives for drug users who continue to use drugs.

HIV/AIDS-related issues constitute a major workload for PHDs. Local strategy to prevent the transmission of HIV is formulated by an AIDS standing committee which all health boards have a statutory responsibility to convene and a multidisciplinary drug action team in which local authorities, police and health boards all cooperate. A balance between primary prevention and harm reduction has to be maintained. Strategy is therefore aimed at maintaining the awareness of the general public, particularly young people, about the risk of HIV and empowering them to adopt behaviours which reduce that risk. In addition, vulnerable groups must be targeted, especially men who have sex with men and intravenous drug users. Preventive services must be made available, e.g. accessible genitourinary medicine services, condom provision, needle exchange and substitute prescribing. Local strategy also encompasses the provision of services for the continuing care, support and treatment of those already affected.

Hepatitis B and the more recently identified hepatitis C viruses are also significant public health issues. Transmission mechanisms for these hepatitis viruses are broadly similar to HIV. Therefore, control of infection measures which have been established to prevent transmission of HIV are equally applicable to hepatitis B and C. Health promotion initiatives and care and treatment provision now have to encompass the broader concept of bloodborne viruses in general rather than concentrating only on HIV.

Bloodborne virus prevention, care and treatment is coordinated by PHDs but is very much a multidisciplinary function. It is a prime example of the importance of cooperation between PHDs, health promotion services, primary and secondary care services, local authorities, police and voluntary agencies.

CONCLUSION

The role of the public health department in the control of communicable disease has evolved over centuries. Many milestones have been achieved, such as:

- the understanding of the principles of the transmission of infection;
- the importance of good hygiene standards in hospitals;
- the discovery of artificially created acquired immunity by immunisation;
- the importance of hand hygiene as a basic infection control measure;
- the importance of food hygiene standards.

The understanding of the epidemiology of communicable disease plays a key role in recognising risk factors for infection. This enables prevention and control measures to be introduced and forms the foundations of the legislation, strategies and policies encompassing communicable disease control.

Although there has been a decline in the mortality associated with communicable diseases, morbidity remains a concern. Increasingly, infection-related issues are being highlighted in the media, raising awareness and concern in both health professionals and the general public. This was particularly apparent at the time of the central Scotland *E. coli* O157 outbreak but has also been demonstrated in the public response to reporting of evolving multidrug-resistant bacteria.

These issues, along with the growing range of health-care services being provided in the community setting, as opposed to hospitals, have raised awareness of infection risks. This has prompted PHDs to acknowledge the need for a wider range of expertise within their communicable disease teams. To enable them to respond to the need for practical infection control guidance in the wider community, many have appointed infection control nurses. The developing PHICN role offers both stimulating and exciting opportunities to improve infection control standards and reduce the risk of infection to patients, health-care staff and the wider community.

Acknowledgement

E. coli O157 epidemiological data and figures used with permission from Dr D Moir, Director of Public Health, Lanarkshire Health Board.

REFERENCES

Caddow P 1989 Applied microbiology. Scutari Press, Harrow
Cooke R 1993 Surgery strategy to thwart bugs. Practice Nurse Feb 15–28: 717–721
Department of Health 1995 Hospital infection control: guidance on the control of infection in hospitals. BAPS, Heywood
Department of Health 1997 Health advice for travellers. DoH, Wetherby
Department of Health and Social Security 1976 Prevention and health: everbody's business – a reassessment of public and personal health. HMSO, London
Department of Health, Welsh Office, Scottish Office Department of Health, DHSS (Northern Ireland) with the Public Health Laboratory Service Communicable Disease Surveillance Centre 1995 Health information for overseas travel. HMSO, London
Department of Health, Welsh Office, Scottish Office Department of Health, DHSS (Northern Ireland) 1996a Immunisation against infectious diseases. HMSO, London
Department of Health and Welsh Office Interdepartmental Working Group on Tuberculosis 1996b The prevention and control of tuberculosis in the United Kingdom: recommendations for the prevention and control of tuberculosis at local level. DoH, Wetherby
Donaldson R J, Donaldson L J 1993 Essential public health medicine. Cromwell, Melksham
Duckworth G, Heathcock R 1995 Report of a combined Working Party of the British Society for Antimicrobial Chemotherapy and the Hospital Infection Society: guidelines on the control of methicillin-resistant *Staphylococcus aureus* in the community, Journal of Hospital Infection 31: 1–12
Hospital Infection Working Group of the Department of Health and the Public Health Laboratory Service 1995 Hospital infection control: guidance on the control of infection in hospitals, DoH, London
Lalonde M 1974 A new perspective on the health of Canadians. Ministry of Supply and Service, Ottawa, Canada
Meers P, Jacobsen W, McPherson M 1992 Hospital infection control for nurses. Chapman and Hall, London

Monto A S, Higashi G I, Marrs C F 1991 Infectious agents. In: Holland W W, Detels R, Knox G (eds) Oxford textbook of public health, vol 1. influences on public health, 2nd edn. Oxford Medical, Oxford

Morgan D R, Lamont T J, Dawson J D, Booth C 1990 Decontamination of instruments and control of cross infection in general practice. British Medical Journal 300: 1379–1380

National Health Service Management Executive 1996 Report of the Short Life Working Group on the Roles and Responsibilities of Health Boards: commissioning better health. NHS MEL (1996) 45. Scottish Office Department of Health, Edinburgh

Pennington Group 1997 Report on the circumstances leading to the 1996 outbreak of infection with *E. coli* O157 in Central Scotland, the implications for food safety and the lessons to be learned. The Stationery Office, Edinburgh

Public Health Medicine Environmental Group 1996 Guidelines on the control of infection in residential and nursing homes. HMSO, London

Richards C, Whitfield L 1995 Travel clinics. The immunisation in general practice series, vol 1. Reed Healthcare Communications, Sutton

Rontree P M, Beard M A 1968 Hospital strains of *Staphylococcus aureus* with particular reference to methicillin resistant strains. Medical Journal of Australia 2: 1163

Scottish Home and Health Department Report of Ministerial Task Force 1992 HIV and AIDS in Scotland: Prevention the key. SOHHD, Edinburgh

Scottish Executive 1999 Review of the public health function in Scotland. SE, Edinburgh

Scottish Office Department of Health 1996 Commissioning better health: Report of the Short Life Working Party on the Roles and Responsibilities of Health Boards. NHS MEL (1996) 45. SODH, Edinburgh

Scottish Office Department of Health 1997 Designed to care: renewing the National Health Service in Scotland. SODH, Edinburgh

Scottish Office Department of Health 1999 Hospital aquired infection: a framework for a national system of surveillance for the NHS in Scotland. SODH, Edinburgh

Scottish Office Department of Health Advisory Group on Infection 1996 The investigation and control of outbreaks of foodborne disease in Scotland. SODH, Edinburgh

Scottish Office Department of Health Advisory Group on Infection 1998 Scottish infection manual. Public Health Policy Unit, Edinburgh

Scottish Office Home and Health Department Report of Ministerial Task Force 1994 Drugs in Scotland: meeting the challenge. SOHHD, Edinburgh

SHAIR group 1995 HIV prevention initiatives in Scotland. Health Education Board for Scotland, Edinburgh

Sneddon J, Ahmed S, Duncan E 1997 Control of infection: a survey of general medical practices. Journal of Public Health Medicine 19(3): 313–319

Strausbaugh L J, Jacobson C, Yost T 1993 Methicillin resistant *Staphylococcus aureus* in a nursing home and affiliated hospital: a four year perspective. Infection Control and Hospital Epidemiology 14(6): 331–336

Tannahill A 1985 What is health promotion? Health Education Journal 44 (4): 167–168

Tones B K 1986 Health education and the ideology of health promotion: a review of alternative approaches. Health Education and Research – Theory and Practice 1(1): 3–12

World Health Organisation 1978 Alma-Ata: primary healthcare. WHO, Geneva

Worsley M A 1998 The role of the infection control nurse. Journal of Hospital Infection 11 (suppl A): 400–405

10

Screening as a disease prevention strategy

Susie Stewart

The preventive health services of modern society fight the battle over a wider front and therefore less dramatically than is the case with personal medicine. Yet the victories won by preventive medicine are much the most important for mankind. This is not so only because it is obviously preferable to prevent suffering rather than alleviate it. Preventive medicine, which is merely another way of saying collective action, builds up a system of social habits that constitute an indispensable part of what we mean by civilisation. (Nye Bevan)

INTRODUCTION

The concept of screening as a strategy for preventing disease – that is, actively seeking to identify a disease or predisease condition in people who are presumed and presume themselves to be healthy – is now widely accepted in health care.

Screening differs from traditional 'curative' medicine because it seeks to detect disease before symptoms present and before an individual decides to seek medical advice. It thus carries a particular ethical responsibility because it contains the potential to move individuals from a state of supposing themselves to be healthy to the state of having some disorder or disease.

It is therefore essential for the health system to be rigorous in evaluating screening programmes or proposals – whether they have been running for many years, as is the case with the national cervical screening programme for women over the age of 20 years, or whether they are being suggested for introduction in the health service today.

It must also be stressed that, ethically, screening should not be used to identify conditions that are either untreatable or insignificant since 'at either end of this spectrum lie anguish and anxiety' (Holland & Stewart 1990).

As Wald & Cuckle (1989) emphasised: 'Screening must be principally concerned with the prevention of disease and the recognition that it is only worthwhile screening for disorders that lend themselves to effective intervention.'

This may sound simple and obvious but it is by no means always the case, although it is central to the integrity of the whole screening process.

Opinions among health professionals on the value of screening remain varied. For example, in the South-East London Screening Study – the only British randomised controlled trial of general health screening in a general practice population – it was found that such screening increased the work of general practitioners by 10% without any corresponding benefit in health terms. The authors concluded:

Any form of screening, including multiphasic, must be judged on the basis of its demonstrable health benefits. Since these control trial results have failed to demonstrate any beneficial effect on either mortality or morbidity, we believe that the use of general proactive based multiphasic screening in the middle-aged can no longer be advocated on scientific, ethical or economic grounds as a desirable public health measure. (South-East London Screening Study Group 1977)

Enthusiasts point to the potential for reducing illness and death. There has been a growth in private screening clinics offering general health-screening programmes for both men and women. And despite the evidence already quoted, there is an increasing emphasis on opportunistic screening in primary care with 'lifestyle' checks for new patients, targets for patients' uptake of screening for cervical cancer and screening for risk of cardiovascular disease in men and women. It is important to highlight the difference between screening where groups of people are invited to be tested and opportunistic screening where the patient has initiated the health contact for some other reason and the opportunity is taken to suggest various other tests appropriate to the patient's age group, such as the measurement of blood pressure in the middle aged.

One fundamental dilemma, raised more than 30 years ago (Nuffield Provincial Hospitals Trust 1968), which is even more relevant today, is that of enthusiastic clinicians, patients and pressure groups, assisted by the media, leading a crusade for the provision of a screening service for a particular disease or group of diseases before a comprehensive and scientifically respectable assessment of benefit and risk is available. There is almost a feeling that if individuals are screened all will be well. This is a damaging and dangerous fallacy.

Opponents of screening cite the harm it can do in terms of misuse of limited health resources, misdiagnosis – either positive or negative – overtreatment and anxiety.

Skrabanek (1988), for example, held the view that 'Screening healthy people without informing them about the magnitude of the inherent risks of screening is ethically unjustifiable'. The possibility that screening may be harmful is often ignored on the assumption that its outcome must be either benefit or no effect. But the results of a study of screening healthy adults for risk of coronary heart disease found that participants did show a significant increase in psychological distress (Stoate 1989) and there have been instances of bowel perforation in colonoscopy screening.

Current opinion on screening for the prevention of disease seems to lie somewhere between the extremes of enthusiasm and doubt in supporting a cautious and scientifically rigorous approach to screening procedures and proposals. But with the fast development of techniques for genetic screening, it is ever more important to examine any proposals for national screening programmes carefully and critically before rather than after they are introduced. And in view of the explosion in demand for health care of all sorts, cost considerations cannot be ignored.

DEFINITIONS

The United States Commission on Chronic Illness (1957) defined screening in the following terms.

Screening is the presumptive identification of unrecognised disease or defect by the application of tests, examinations, or other procedures which can be applied rapidly. Screening tests sort out apparently well persons who apparently have a disease from those who probably do not. A screening test is not intended to be diagnostic. Persons with positive or suspicious findings must be referred to their physicians for diagnosis and necessary treatment.

This particular definition is couched in strikingly defensive terms. In the United States law suits have been filed against physicians who have failed to detect cancer, among other diseases, on screening and medical litigation has increased markedly in recent years. The same is beginning to happen in the United Kingdom.

Wilson & Jungner (1968), in their milestone document for the World Health Organisation, differentiated various types of screening, as laid out in Table 10.1.

A simple working definition of screening is shown in Box 10.1 and provides a useful general explanation of the process for practical purposes (Stone & Stewart 1994).

BENEFITS AND DISADVANTAGES OF SCREENING

Screening presents as an attractive proposition because it seems to offer the opportunity to advance the clinical horizon of presymptomatic disease, to achieve earlier diagnosis and thereby to improve prognosis.

Chamberlain (1984) summarised the benefits and disadvantages of screening as shown in Box 10.2.

The benefits are clear. Some of those identified will have a better prognosis because of early diagnosis and treatment. Disease diagnosed earlier may

Table 10.1 Types of screening

Type of screening	Description
Mass screening	Large-scale screening of whole population groups
Selective screening	Screening of selected high-risk groups in the community
Multiphasic screening	Administration of two or more screening tests to large groups of people
Surveillance	Long-term observation of individuals or populations
Case finding	Screening of patients already in contact with the health services for the purpose of detecting and treating disease
Opportunistic screening	When opportunity is taken at a routine consultation – for example, with a GP or practice nurse – to ask about health-related behaviour

Box 10.1

Screening is a preventive activity which seeks to identify an unsuspected disease or predisease condition for which an effective intervention is available.

Box 10.2 Benefits and disadvantages of screening

Benefits	Disadvantages
Improved prognosis for some cases detected	Longer morbidity for cases whose prognosis is unaltered
Less radical treatment which cures some early cases	Overtreatment of questionable abnormalities
Resource savings	Resource costs
Reassurance for those with negative test results	False reassurance for those with false-negative results
	Anxiety and sometimes morbidity for those with false-positive results
	Hazard from screening test itself

respond to less radical treatment. There should be savings in terms of health service resources by treating diseases before they progress. Those with true-negative results can be reassured.

The disadvantages of screening are less obvious. They include longer periods of illness in patients whose prognosis is unaltered in spite of early diagnosis. And there can be overtreatment of insignificant conditions or minor abnormalities. Haynes et al (1978), in a randomised study of steelworkers with raised diastolic pressure, found that absenteeism from work increased after they had been told they had hypertension. There are resource costs involved in identifying more illness – the costs of the screening tests themselves and of subsequent treatment or management of whatever is diagnosed and the manpower costs.

There are also the two gremlins of false-negative and false-positive results as defined in Box 10.3.

Of course, false positives and false negatives occur in all diagnostic

Box 10.3	
False negatives	When tests seem to show that people do not have a disease or condition when in fact they do
False positives	When tests seem to show that people do have a disease or condition when in fact they do not

tests. But they are more prominent in the screening process because of the greater numbers being tested in one screening programme and because in most instances the screening has been initiated by the system rather than the individual. These failures are serious because they lead to false reassurance for individuals who are told wrongly they do not have the disease being screened for – as illustrated distressingly, for example, in mistakes in the reading of cervical smears in recent times. And they also cause at least anxiety and sometimes actual illness in individuals who are recalled unnecessarily for further tests when they do not have the disease. Finally, there is the possibility of the screening test itself causing harm as, for example, in the early days of amniocentesis where there was a small risk of miscarriage.

PRINCIPLES UPON WHICH SCREENING SHOULD BE BASED

It is thus clear that screening is not a procedure that should be lightly undertaken. As Berwick observed in 1985: 'The mere existence of unrecognised cases of illness is, by itself, insufficient reason to screen. Disease has many faces, and the hunt is not benign'.

During the 1960s, there was a surge of enthusiasm for screening as a result in part of improved diagnostic techniques and methods of analysis. The World Health Organisation then invited Wilson & Jungner to produce a set of guidelines and principles upon which any worthwhile screening programme should be based. These were published in 1968 and are reproduced as Box 10.4.

In 1984 Cuckle & Wald summarised the basic requirements of a screening programme under eight headings (Table 10.2).

In 1990 Holland & Stewart grouped the screening principles into the four categories of condition, diagnosis, treatment and cost (Box 10.5).

The basic principles of screening remain valid but society has changed 30 years after their original publication and there are those who feel they need to be redefined to meet current conditions.

In the United Kingdom, the Department of Health has now set up a National Screening Committee to develop updated principles for appraisal of proposed screening programmes and this will be covered in more detail later in the chapter.

Box 10.4   Wilson & Jungner's (1968) principles of screening

The condition sought should be an important health problem.
There should be an accepted treatment for patients with recognised disease.
Facilities for diagnosis and treatment should be available.
There should be a recognisable latent or early symptomatic stage.
There should be a suitable test or examination.
The test should be acceptable to the population.
The natural history of the disease, including latent to declared disease, should be adequately understood.
There should be an agreed policy on whom to treat as patients.
The cost of case finding (including diagnosis and treatment of patients diagnosed) should be economically balanced in relation to possible expenditure on medical care as a whole.
Case finding should be a continuing process and not a 'once-for-all' project.

Table 10.2   Requirements for a worthwhile screening programme

Aspect	Requirement
Disorder	Well defined
Prevalence	Known
Natural history	Mentally important disorder for which there is an effective remedy available
Financial	Cost effective
Facilities	Available or easily installed
Ethical	Procedures following a positive result are generally agreed and acceptable both to the screening authorities and to the patients
Test	Simple and safe
Test performance	Distributions of test values in affected and unaffected individuals known, extent of overlap sufficiently small and suitable cut-off level defined

---

Box 10.5   Screening principles of condition, diagnosis, treatment and cost

Condition	Condition sought should be an important health problem whose natural history, including development from latent to declared disease, is adequately understood. The condition should have a recognisable latent or early symptomatic stage.
Diagnosis	There should be a suitable diagnostic test which is available, safe and acceptable to the population concerned. There should be an agreed policy, based on test findings and national standards, as to whom to regard as patients and the whole process should be a continuing one.
Treatment	There should be an accepted and proven treatment or intervention for patients identified as having the disease or predisease condition and facilities for treatment should be available.
Cost	The cost of case finding (including diagnosis and treatment) should be economically balanced in relation to possible expenditure on medical care as a whole.

Muir Gray (1997), who is a member of the National Committee, has suggested that the original criteria are weak in the following ways.

- There is insufficient emphasis on the adverse effects of screening and the need to ensure that a programme does more good than harm. Although these factors were important in the 1960s, in the context of a better informed, more assertive public, which is more likely to sue if harm is done, it is essential to concentrate on these factors.
- The criteria state that an 'accepted treatment' should be available but many accepted treatments are either ineffective or of unproven efficacy.
- There is no discussion of the quality of the evidence upon which the decision should be made.

CRITERIA FOR THE EVALUATION OF SCREENING

Evaluation is of critical importance in screening and has too often been neglected in the establishment of screening programmes. In 1971 Cochrane & Holland wrote:

We believe there is an ethical difference between everyday medical practice and screening. If a patient asks a medical practitioner for help, the doctor does the best he can. He is not responsible for defects in medical knowledge. If, however, the practitioner initiates screening procedures he is in a very different situation. He should, in our view, have conclusive evidence that screening can alter the natural history of the disease in a significant proportion of those screened.

Cochrane & Holland (1971) suggested seven criteria for the assessment and evaluation of any screening test, which remain valid today and are as follows.

1. *Simplicity* – a test should be simple to perform, easy to interpret and, where possible, capable of use by nurses and other paramedical personnel.
2. *Acceptability* – since participation in screening is voluntary, a test must be acceptable to those being invited to undergo it.
3. *Accuracy* – a test must give a true measurement of the condition or symptom under investigation.
4. *Cost* – the expense of the test must be considered in relation to the benefits of early detection of the disease.
5. *Repeatability* – the test should give consistent results in repeated trials.
6. *Sensitivity* – the test should be capable of giving a positive finding when the individual being screened has the disease being sought.
7. *Specificity* – the test should be capable of giving a negative finding when the person being screened does not have the disease being sought.

One of the main criticisms of screening has been that tests have often been used without accurate knowledge of their scope and limitations. In the early days, matters were much simpler. The natural history of conditions being screened for, such as tuberculosis and syphilis, was well understood, as were the appropriate lines of treatment.

The emphasis now is on the chronic diseases about which much less is known and the area of uncertainty is greatest in those conditions which take many years to develop and in which there is no clear boundary between the healthy and the diseased. (Wilson 1963)

SCREENING IN PRACTICE

So, in practical terms, where are we in relation to screening in the United Kingdom at the beginning of the 21st century?

National Screening Committee

The establishment of the National Screening Committee (NSC) in 1996 was a welcome, if long overdue, government initiative. Its initial aim was to review the whole of screening – a massive task – and to identify key issues such as ethical considerations and to confirm criteria to be met before the introduction of new programmes. The main role of the Committee is to advise on:

- the case for implementing new population screening programmes not presently purchased by the NHS;
- implementing screening technologies of proven effectiveness but which require controlled and well-managed introduction;
- the case for continuing, modifying or withdrawing existing population screening programmes, in particular programmes inadequately evaluated or of doubtful effectiveness, quality or value.

The Committee's national inventory of screening identified over 300 screening programmes, many still at the research stage, many others introduced locally to meet various local needs and adhering to individual local arrangements and protocols. One frequent criticism of the state of screening in the UK is that the availability and certainly the quality of many screening procedures can depend to an unacceptable extent on where an individual happens to live, with considerable variation in different parts of the country. There must be a consistent and reliable approach to screening regardless of locality and the NSC now has the formidable task of assessing which existing programmes meet its strict criteria.

A framework for screening

The NSC has set out a framework for screening using many of the concepts, principles and criteria described earlier in the chapter. This begins by defining screening as:

'...the systematic application of a test or inquiry, to identify individuals at sufficient risk of a specific disorder to warrant further investigation or direct preventive action, amongst people who have not sought medical attention on account of symptoms of that disorder.'

Screening can be either *proactive* – when members of a target population are invited to attend for testing in a systematic programme which will cover the whole of that population in a defined period of time – or *opportunistic* – when an individual is offered a test for an unsuspected disorder when visiting the doctor for another reason.

The NSC (1998) has set out criteria for appraising the viability, effectiveness and appropriateness of a screening programme. As will be seen, the criteria are based on the classic criteria previously described but take into account both the more rigorous standards or evidence required to improve effectiveness and the greater concern about the adverse effects of health care.

The NSC criteria for screening are as follows.

The condition

- The condition should be an important health problem.
- The epidemiology and natural history of the condition, including development from latent to declared disease, should be adequately understood and there should be a detectable risk factor, disease marker, latent period or early symptomatic stage.
- All the cost-effective primary prevention interventions should have been implemented as far as practicable.

The test

- There should be a simple, safe, precise and validated screening test.
- The distribution of test values in the target population should be known and a suitable cut-off level defined and agreed.
- The test should be acceptable to the population.
- There should be an agreed policy on the further diagnostic investigation of individuals with a positive test result and on the choices available to those individuals.

The treatment

- There should be an effective treatment or intervention for patients identified through early detection, with evidence of early treatment leading to better outcomes than late treatment.
- There should be agreed evidence-based policies covering which individuals should be offered treatment and the appropriate treatment to be offered.

- Clinical management of the condition and patient outcomes should be optimised by all health-care providers prior to participation in a screening programme.

The screening programme

- There should be evidence from high-quality randomised controlled trials that the screening programme is effective in reducing mortality or morbidity.
- There should be evidence that the complete screening programme (test, diagnostic procedures, treatment/intervention) is clinically, socially and ethically acceptable to health professionals and the public.
- The benefit from the screening programme should outweigh the physical and psychological harm (caused by the test, diagnostic procedures and treatment).
- The opportunity cost of the screening programme (including testing, diagnosis and treatment) should be economically balanced in relation to expenditure on medical care as a whole.
- There should be a plan for managing and monitoring the screening programme and an agreed set of quality assurance standards.
- Adequate staffing and facilities for testing, diagnosis, treatment and programme management should be available prior to the commencement of the screening programme.
- All other options for managing the condition should have been considered – for example, improving treatment, providing other services.

These criteria are exceedingly stringent and rightly so and have probably not been met in any screening programme so far introduced.

Current state of national screening programmes in the UK

There are the existing national screening programmes for women for breast and cervical cancer and there are those who feel that there should be equivalent national programmes for men in terms, for example, of prostatic cancer. There are routine procedures for screening in infancy and childhood, some of which are of undoubted value and others which may be more questionable in their effectiveness. There is the exploding area of genetic screening which promises a Pandora's box of ethical and social dilemmas. And there is the important area of opportunistic screening in primary care, of value particularly perhaps in adolescents of both sexes and middle-aged men, where a consultation for a specific purpose in relatively inaccessible patient groups can provide an opportunity to screen, and in the elderly who may have undetected problems – for example, defective hearing or sight or social isolation – whose identification can make a huge difference to their quality of life.

Screening for cervical cancer

It has been claimed that most cervical cancers could be prevented or effectively treated if all women were offered and complied with high-quality cytological screening programmes (Berrino 1988). To this end a national cervical screening programme was established in the UK in 1964. The current policy remains to screen women aged between 25 and 64 years (20 and 60 years in Scotland) at least every 5 years.

Results of a collaborative study of 10 screening programmes in eight countries (IARC 1986) suggested that screening should be aimed mainly at women aged 35–60 but should begin some years before age 35 and that intervals between screens should ideally be 3 years or less.

The Imperial Cancer Research Fund Coordinating Committee suggested seven basic requirements for a successful cervical screening programme.

1. Satisfactory resources for taking, examining and reporting on smears.
2. Acceptable arrangements for making and keeping appointments for examination.
3. Acceptable arrangements for actual taking of smears.
4. Accurate listing of women in target population to enable complete initial call of eligible women and ensure regular recall as appropriate.
5. An informed client population who know and understand the function of the procedure.
6. Continuing scrutiny of records to ensure appropriate follow-up.
7. Ability to monitor efficiency and effectiveness of the programme and to adjust policies and procedures accordingly.

In the UK, the national programme has not yet produced the expected reduction in mortality (Roberts 1989, Murphy et al 1988). It is generally felt that this has related mainly to organisation, accountability and commitment rather than to finance or expertise (Roberts 1989, Richards 1985), although there have been some well-publicised and tragic failures of the programme.

It has been suggested that the most successful cervical screening programmes have three main elements in common (Editorial 1985). First, they are organised as public health, cancer control programmes with the specific objective of reducing mortality. Second, they concentrate first on the never screened and on the age groups at greatest risk and they persist. Third, and absolutely crucial, there is a specific individual in charge of screening who is responsible and accountable for the programme.

In general, cervical screening seems to be most effectively based around general practice although in certain areas, such as deprived inner cities, and among certain minority groups, a different approach may be more successful. The general practitioner is in a good position to offer information and reassurance about the tests, especially to older women who no longer attend child or family planning clinics (Havelock et al 1988). The results also come direct to the general practitioner to be filed in the patient's records and so are readily accessible (Ross 1989).

In one study of cervical screening in general practice, an uptake rate of 96% was achieved (Standing & Mercer 1984). The authors acknowledge that this was helped by having a relatively stable patient list, most of whom were known to the doctor. In this practice in a compact urban setting, the nurses backed up by the general practitioner worked best for effective screening.

The National Audit Office (1998) has recently published a report on *The performance of the NHS cervical screening programme in England*. It concludes that although improvements have been made, considerable scope remains for improving the service that women receive and pinpoints in particular the serious failings in the quality of the interpretation and reporting of smears at a small number of laboratories. Recent steps have been taken by the NHS Executive and external accreditation of screening laboratories is now mandatory.

Screening for breast cancer

Breast cancer is the most common form of cancer among women in the UK and the Scottish mortality rates are among the highest in the world.

The NHS breast cancer screening programme was set up in 1988 and invites women aged 50–64 years for screening every 3 years. Women over the upper age limit can request screening but will not be called automatically. Trials on the appropriateness of the lower age limit are under way but results are not yet available.

The Forrest Working Group (1986), on whose recommendations the national programme was established, suggested six requirements for the organisation of a breast cancer screening programme.

1. Women in the target group should be sent a personal invitation from their general practitioner.
2. Arrangements for recording positive results at the basic screen must include a fail-safe mechanism to ensure that action is taken on all positive results.
3. Every basic screening unit should have access to a specialist team for the assessment of screen-detected abnormalities.
4. A screening record system should be developed to identify, invite and recall women eligible for screening; to record attendance for screening and results; and to monitor the screening process and its effectiveness.
5. There should be adequate arrangements for quality control both within and between centres so that an acceptable standard of mammography can be maintained.
6. A designated person should be responsible for managing each local screening service. The person chosen would have managerial ability and is likely to have experience in community or preventive health care, although the radiological aspects must be the responsibility of a consultant radiologist.

Those charged with establishing the programme were determined to avoid the problems associated with the long-established cervical screening programme. Two fundamental problems, however, surround the concept of screening for breast cancer. In the first place, although much is known about the aetiology of the condition, it is still not possible to prevent it. And in the second place, although early diagnosis improves prognosis, available treatment is not satisfactory since about two-thirds of those with the disease are likely to die from it sooner or later.

The programme, which is very much nurse run, is now well established and appears to be working smoothly with a satisfactory response rate. Results of a Finnish population-based cohort study (Hakama et al 1997) suggest that a breast-screening programme can achieve a similar effect on mortality as achieved in scientific trials but that current programmes have yet to show any unequivocal benefit in terms of either mortality or life-years.

And of course, mortality is not the only endpoint from a human perspective; no one has yet adequately measured the disadvantages of screening for breast cancer, particularly in view of the high number of false-positive results produced in trials so far. A Swedish study of false-positive findings (Lidbrink et al 1996) concludes: 'The examinations and investigations carried out after false-positive mammography – especially in women under 50 – and the cost of these procedures are a neglected but substantial problem'.

There is still considerable discussion about whether screening is the best use of scarce resources in this particular condition. In 1989 Maureen Roberts, one of the pioneers behind the research which led to the establishment of the programme, herself posed the question as to whether this was the right way to provide the best possible benefit for women. Screening is always a second best, an admission of the failure of prevention or treatment, and perhaps resources currently devoted to screening would be better used for research into effective treatment.

Apart from a number of well-established screening procedures in the antenatal and neonatal period, these are the only two national screening programmes in this country at the present time. There are those who believe that there should be an equivalent screening programme for cancer of the prostate in adult men, for ovarian cancer in women and for colorectal cancer.

Screening for prostate cancer

Cancer of the prostate is rare in men below the age of 50 years but results of the first large-scale randomised trial suggest that routine screening for prostate cancer would significantly reduce mortality. The leader of this Canadian trial favours starting measurements of prostate-specific antigen (PSA) 'annually at the age of 50 years in the general population and at 40 years for those at high risk – namely, those with a familial history of prostate cancer and black Americans'. Men with abnormal PSA could then be recalled for further tests. Critics of the study point out that only 23% of 30 000 men invited for screening accepted and suggest that further research is needed.

In the UK, screening for this condition has been examined by the NSC who concluded, on the basis of two systematic reviews specially commissioned, that it should not be provided by the NHS or offered to the public until there is new evidence of an effective screening technology. Current technologies have a limited accuracy that could lead to a positive result in those without the disease and follow-up procedures could cause unnecessary harm to healthy individuals. The NSC will keep emerging research on this under review.

Screening for colorectal cancer

Colorectal cancer is a major public health problem and the second most common cause of cancer deaths in the UK. The NSC recommended two pilot studies of screening which started in 1999 and will run for 2 years. During the pilot phase, preparatory planning work will take place to allow rapid implementation of a national screening programme should the results indicate that screening does more good than harm at a reasonable cost. A central feature of the pilot studies will be the provision of clear and explicit information to people invited for screening not only about the benefits of colorectal cancer screening but also about its adverse effects and limitations.

Screening in infancy

Infancy, particularly in the neonatal period, is a time of life when certain screening procedures are routinely carried out. Two examples of routine procedures illustrate the central harm-versus-benefit dilemma of screening.

The first – screening for phenylketonuria (PKU) and hypothyroidism by routine Guthrie testing – is simple and undoubtedly advantageous; the other – screening for congenital dislocation of the hip (CDH) – is still the subject of considerable debate.

Testing for PKU is the most accepted form of neonatal screening in the European Union. The birth prevalence of the condition is around 11 per 100 000 babies screened although there are variations within and between countries. The condition is a prime candidate for screening and satisfies most if not all the criteria for a population programme.

It is an important health problem. If untreated, it has serious consequences, the most important of which is progressive mental retardation often with associated neurological damage. The mechanics of the condition are well understood, there is a suitable diagnostic test which is available, safe and acceptable to the population, and treatment is successful. The Guthrie blood test is performed routinely in the UK between the sixth and 10th days of life and is a satisfactory and sensitive method. PKU also satisfies the treatment principle as it can be very effectively treated, essentially by diet. It also seems reasonable to accept that screening is cost effective since the prevention of severe mental retardation releases the community and the health service from the need to provide long-term medical and social supervision. That few people today have seen a case of untreated classic PKU in a young child is a testament to the success of the screening programme for this condition. The fact that babies can be tested for hypothyroidism from the same sample, with all the benefits of early treatment that confers, gives added value to this simple screening test.

Screening for congenital dislocation of the hip – one of the most common congenital defects of the locomotor system – is altogether more controversial. Leck (1986) summarised four main problem areas in screening for this condition as currently practised. The first concerns false-positive results. Most screened cases in which unstable hips are reported are false positives, at least in the sense that they would not progress to dislocation if left untreated. There is thus a risk of overtreatment.

The second problem relates to false-negative results which occur in roughly the same proportion as false positives. It is not known how often in these false-negative cases instability was in fact present but missed in neonatal screening and how often it genuinely develops later.

The third problem area concerns treatment policies where there is disagreement among experts about the indications for and the methods and duration of treatment. And finally there remains considerable doubt about the outcome of early treatment.

An editorial in the *British Medical Journal* (1998) underlines the confusion surrounding screening for CDH.

The Ortolani or Barlow test for hip instability has been universally used in Britain for 30 years. It fails to identify two-thirds of the hips which subsequently need surgical treatment and has made little or no difference to the number coming for surgery. It causes many infants to be splinted who probably have no hip disorder.

FORWARD PLAN

Over the next three years, the National Screening Committee will develop the screening aspects of the National Service Frameworks for Diabetes, Coronary Heart Disease and Health in Old Age. It will also develop work on its recommendations on antenatal and childhood screening as well as considering emerging research on screening for prostate cancer and ovarian cancer. Issues of informed choice, genetic screening, and access to screening for people from ethnic minorities and people with learning disabilities are also being considered.

CONCLUSION

The dark side of medicine – the harm that medical care can do – has been mentioned earlier in the chapter and was highlighted more than 20 years ago by Illich (1975). He warned that harm can go beyond the side-effects of drugs or inappropriate use of high-intensity treatment to the social and psychological consequences of unchecked medicalisation of some aspects of modern life. This warning has been reiterated recently by Porter (1997) who asserts that the healthier Western society becomes, the more medicine it craves and that doctors and consumers are becoming locked into a fantasy that all people have something wrong with them and everything can be cured. There are those who would argue in favour of an urgent debate about the fundamental issue of the meaning of health and health care and the need to redefine consumer expectations and whether it may be time to establish an Illich Collaboration to make readily available objective evidence of harms of medical care (Edwards 1999).

In view of this kind of thinking and of the growing demands for health care, increasingly complex medical technologies, a spreading appetite for litigation and the inevitability of some form of rationing in whatever disguise, it is ever more imperative to look critically and in a national context at population screening as an effective strategy for prevention.

The organisation of screening on the ground must also be rigorously scrutinised. The Public Accounts Committee Report on the performance of the Cervical Screening Programme in England, published in December 1998, warned that lives remain at risk because there are still 'worrying failures at every stage of the cervical screening programme'. And one of the architects of the national screening programme for breast cancer set up in 1987, Professor Michael Baum, has recently stated that 'Today I believe that breast screening may not be the best use of scarce NHS resources available to combat this disease'. He points out that the screening programme, which costs £35 million a year to run, 'is limiting funds for the introduction of new drug treatments which is where the real hope for conquering breast cancer lies'.

Of course, hindsight is a powerful tool but questions do need to be asked about the best use of resources in screening, as in other areas of the health service. Perceptions of health and health care have to change as circumstances change – as they have done perceptibly in the 50 years since the establishment of the NHS. To appreciate the truth of this, one has only to consider Beveridge's understandable but naïve vision of a 'health service which will diminish disease by prevention and cure' (Watkin 1975).

A flexibility of focus for all health professionals is essential if success in improving the health of the population as a whole is to be gradually achieved. Government, health professionals and the public must acknowledge two distinct strands in any health-care system – health care, which provides for those who are ill, and health gain or health improvement, which strives to produce better health at a population level.

There is already growing acceptance that the strictly medical model of health is fatally flawed, that health is multidimensional and that while health care is essential it should not be allowed to dominate the health policy agenda to the exclusion of other key factors that contribute to health improvement.

A population approach to health is a difficult concept to achieve in a society where the focus has traditionally been very much on the individual:

Everyone says that prevention is better than cure and hardly anyone acts as if they believe it ... Palliatives nearly always take precedence over prevention ...
Treatment – the attempt to cure the sick – is more tangible, more exciting and more immediately rewarding than prevention. (Mackintosh 1953)

A productive way forward in screening would be threefold.

1. The application of the NSC principles to existing and proposed population screening programmes coupled with a willingness to accept changes to or cessation of existing programmes if necessary, as further scientific evidence becomes available.
2. Screening, with informed consent, for certain high-risk groups such as those with a family history of particular conditions.
3. Opportunistic screening in primary care, with tests which are simple and inexpensive to administer, which could yield quite a harvest of social and minor medical problems the correction of which could make a considerable difference to quality of life.

Screening, carried out in accordance with the strict principles and criteria described in this chapter and subjected to continuing and rigorous evaluation, can become a powerful tool for health improvement.

Acknowledgements

I would like to thank Professor Walter Holland, Dr Grace Lindsay, Dr Lewis Reay, Mr Allan Stewart and Dr David Stone for their constructive comments on the penultimate draft.

REFERENCES

Berrino F 1988 Cervical cancer. In: Silman A J, Allwright S P A (eds) Elimination or reduction of diseases. Oxford University Press, Oxford
Chamberlain J M 1984 Which prescriptive screening services are worthwhile? Journal of Epidemiology and Community Health 38: 270–277
Cochrane A L, Holland W W 1971 Validation of screening procedures. British Medical Bulletin 27(1): 3–8
Cuckle H S, Wald N J 1984 Principles of screening. In: Wald N J (ed) Antenatal and neonatal screening. Oxford University Press, Oxford
Edwards R H T 1999 Is it time for an Illich Collaboration to make available information on the harms of medical care? British Medical Journal 318: 58
Forrest P 1986 Breast cancer screening. Report to the Health Ministers of England, Wales, Scotland and Northern Ireland by a working group chaired by Professor Sir Patrick Forrest. HMSO, London

Hakama M, Pukkala E, Heikkila M, Kallio M 1997 Effectiveness of the public health policy for breast cancer screening in Finland: population based cohort study. British Medical Journal 314: 864

Havelock C M, Webb J, Queenborough J 1988 Preliminary results of a district call scheme for cervical cancer organised in general practice. British Medical Journal 297: 271–275

Haynes R B, Sackett D L, Taylor D W, Gibson E S, Johnson A L 1978 Increased absenteeism from work after detection and labelling of hypertensive patients. New England Journal of Medicine 299: 741–744

Holland W W, Stewart S 1990 Screening in health care: benefit or bane? Nuffield Provincial Hospitals Trust, London

IARC Working Group on Evaluation of Cervical Cancer Screening Programmes 1986 Screening for squamous cervical cancer. British Medical Journal 293: 659–664

Illich I 1975 Medical nemesis: the expropriation of health. Calder and Boyars, London

Leck I 1986 An epidemiological assessment of neonatal screening for dislocation of the hip. Journal of the Royal College of Physicians of London 20: 56–62

Lidbrink E, Elfving J, Frisell J, Jonsson E 1996 Neglected aspects of false positive findings of mammography in breast cancer screening: analysis of false positive cases from the Stockholm trial. British Medical Journal 312: 273–276

Muir Gray J A 1997 Evidence-based healthcare. Churchill Livingstone, Edinburgh

Murphy M F G, Campbell M J, Goldblatt P O 1988 Twenty-years' screening for cancer of the uterine cervix in Great Britain, 1964–1984: further evidence for its ineffectiveness. Journal of Epidemiology and Community Health 42: 49–53

National Audit Office 1998 The performance of the NHS cervical screening programme in England. NAO, London

National Screening Committee 1998 First report of the NSC. Department of Health, London

Nuffield Provincial Hospitals Trust 1968 Screening in medical care: reviewing the evidence. Oxford University Press, Oxford

Porter R 1997 The greatest benefit to mankind: a medical history of humanity from antiquity to the present. Harper Collins, London

Richards T 1985 Poor organisation and lack of will have caused the failure of cervical screening. British Medical Journal 291: 1135

Roberts M M 1989 Breast screening: time for a re-think? British Medical Journal 299: 1153–1155

Ross S K 1989 Cervical cytology screening and government policy. British Medical Journal 299: 101–104

Skrabanek P 1988 The physician's responsibility to the patient. Lancet 1: 1155–1157

South-East London Screening Study Group 1977 A controlled study of multiphasic screening in middle age. International Journal of Epidemiology 6: 357–363

Standing P, Mercer S 1984 Quinquennial cervical smears: every woman's right and every general practitioner's responsibility. British Medical Journal 289: 883–886

Stone D H, Stewart S (eds) 1994 Towards a screening strategy for Scotland. Scottish Forum for Public Health Medicine, Glasgow

US Commission on Chronic Illness 1957 Chronic illness in the United States. Harvard University Press, Cambridge, MA

Wald N, Cuckle H 1989 Reporting the assessment of screening and diagnostic tests. British Journal of Obstetrics and Gynaecology 96: 389–396

Wilson J M G 1963 Multiple screening. Lancet ii: 51–54

Wilson J M G, Jungner G 1968 Principles and practice of screening for disease. World Health Organisation, Geneva

11

Public health in primary care

Pat Turton   Stephen Peckham   Pat Taylor

INTRODUCTION

Primary care is increasingly being considered vital to the promotion of good health and the effective management of health service resources. It is often perceived as being a low-cost alternative to 'high-tech' secondary and tertiary care but although its principles may be simple, the complexity of the social, political and professional context of the development of primary care means that it is often poorly understood and that policies designed to take place in primary care settings are frequently not effectively implemented.

The most recent NHS reforms suggest that primary care should embrace a public health approach, providing the above-mentioned complexities are recognised and dealt with. This chapter introduces models of primary care currently in use and explores the potential for a wider public health model of primary care. It outlines the definitions of primary care and public health and places current practice within a social and historical context. The interface between primary care and public health is explored and examples of practice are provided that highlight the potential benefits to health of integrating primary care and public health models.

THE HISTORICAL CONTEXT OF PRIMARY CARE

It is said that those who do not understand their history are doomed to repeat it, so on that basis, scrutiny of the historical development of health services and primary care in the UK could help us to avoid reinventing old problems.

Klein (1989) noted that the introduction of the NHS on July 5 1948 represented: 'The transformation of an inadequate, partial and muddled patchwork of health care provision into a neat administrative structure'. However, the 'neat administrative structure' largely referred to the hospital sector; primary and community services remained somewhat fragmented and split between a number of agencies. Prior to 1948, primary health care was not referred to as such but community-based medical care was provided either through local government and voluntary organisations or by general practitioners (GPs). Local government provided care ranging from hospital services (from workhouse roots) through to chronic care for the elderly and mentally ill, including maternity and child welfare clinics and services for schoolchildren. Some district (home) nursing services were also provided in the community and public health nurses, in the form of health visitors, were employed by local authorities to work in deprived city areas. Many medical services were not free. For example, in the slums of Glasgow, payment for treatment in the voluntary sector was either by charitable fundraising or by charging those who could afford it, sometimes out of contributory insurance schemes. Chronic cases were regularly discharged from the voluntary hospitals into the care of the municipal authorities. These authorities provided a basic free service to their local poor but would not provide services for those outside their own districts (Webster 1993). Provision was extremely patchy and unequally distributed.

Since 1911, GPs had provided free medical care to those employed patients on their 'panel'. This was limited to manual workers and excluded even their families. Throughout the country, the quality and amount of care available were variable and there was no agreed definition of who should be considered a specialist. In the smaller cottage hospitals, outside the large towns, it was frequently the local GPs who carried out both medical and surgical procedures with no check on their competence to do the job.

During this early period, ordinary community nursing in the United Kingdom was of low status and generally unregulated. Parish councils and local authorities provided some nursing services for the poor. These nurses were frequently, indeed usually, lacking in any formal training. The middle classes employed nurses independently to tend patients in their own homes and to provide midwifery services. Some of these nurses had received some training: for example, the Elizabeth Fry Institute of Nursing had trained nurses for private households from 1840. Some religious orders, particularly in Europe, had a long tradition of providing nursing care to the poor and needy. The voluntary hospitals, of which St Thomas' Hospital in London is a good example, were meanwhile training many more nurses. Some of these women went on to become the first community nurses and early health visitors, in the tradition of the Victorian reformers and charitable workers (Abel-Smith 1960).

Two main themes emerged during the interwar period:

1. a theme which derives from the public health movement and out of which has grown the tradition of public health nursing;
2. a theme which centres around access to health-care services, either via the hospital system directly or else via the general practitioner services.

Between these themes there is a tension which still remains unresolved. They also have a particular relevance for the current development of primary care.

The first theme equates with a public health model emphasising the obligation of public authorities to provide health services for the whole community – a more collectivist approach based on a social model of health. The second theme, around which the Lloyd George insurance scheme was based, emphasised the right of individuals to medical care (based on the purchase of appropriate individual insurance entitlements). A distinction was therefore made between medical care (as in that provided by doctors with the aim of curing illness) and the wider sense of providing the types of care and intervention which would influence the health of the community as a whole.

During the interwar years and subsequently, the dominating influence in health policy development was the increasing medical profession-alisation of public health and the growing power of the royal colleges (i.e. physicians and surgeons). The independence, and hence power and control, of the professions was retained after the introduction of the new NHS, which upheld the dominant professional paradigm and hence the medical model of health-care provision. There was a strong underlying assumption that the provision of better medical care would result in improvement of health overall and a subsequent reduction in the need for health-care services. With hindsight, however, although the importance of efficient and effective provision of curative services is undeniable, this assumption overlooked the effect of wider social and environmental factors on health and health-care needs. These factors could not be addressed by medical services alone.

With regard to primary medical services, after 1948 the previous insurance committees were replaced by executive committees. All GPs were to be in contract with these committees and hence with the NHS. All people were to have the right to be registered with a GP. This latter fundamental right continues to this day and GPs continue to maintain independent contractor status. Since the NHS reforms of 1990, they have considerably widened their role and have become the dominant part of what has come to be known as the 'primary care-led NHS'. However, because of their independent contractor status and medical focus, GPs are considered by many to be somewhat of a barrier to the development of primary care and the integration within it of a public health role.

In this context, we should note a final point in respect of the early years of health service development. This is the role of the local authorities in the provision of public/primary health-care services. These agencies had a key role in the provision of a healthy environment through public health services, such as population screening for TB, and a proactive role with housing and the enforcement of environmental and occupational health regulations. In addition, the provision of local authority health centres as part of primary and community care was a factor in creating environments where professionals might work collaboratively from a joint base. These health centres aimed to develop a holistic model of care and represented a bridge between the medical services and those health services provided by the local authority to the community.

THE CONCEPT OF PRIMARY HEALTH CARE

Primary health care is one of those 'taken for granted' terms which often serves to confuse rather than illuminate. In general, it is taken to refer to health-care issues outside those services provided in a hospital setting. As such, it is clearly socially and culturally defined and in fact, it was not really described as a concept prior to the 1970s. Before that time, in the UK, references were made to individual professions or groups, such as general practitioners, family practitioners, district nurses, health visitors and public health nurses. Services outside hospitals and not part of family doctor services were sometimes referred to as 'community services' or community clinics.

DEFINITIONS AND MODELS OF PRIMARY CARE

Although not referred to as such, the early phase of primary health care was the individual physician in the community providing curative medical services, alongside other individual professionals such as home nurses and midwives, all working independently.

Originating from these roots of general practice and community nursing, the term 'primary health care' first emerged into general usage during the 1970s. Since the major NHS reforms introduced at the end of the 1980s, as outlined in the three White Papers *Promoting better health* (DHSS 1987), *Working for patients* (DoH 1989a) and *Caring for people* (DoH 1989b), the term has been used extensively in the UK. The central organisational structure around which it is based remains the GP practice.

Macdonald (1992) notes that this model configured around the GP services can be regarded as 'primary medical care' and contrasts it with a different and broader primary care approach involving the whole community, such as that outlined by the World Health Organisation, where the focus is on population health as opposed to the health status and treatment of individuals.

A frequently used definition, which in some respect draws these two models together, is that employed by Gamble (1974), who refers to primary care as: 'The care provided at the first point of contact with the health care services'. This definition could in theory cover all those professionals to whom the general public can self-refer and could include, for example, casualty departments, community pharmacists, opticians, dentists and midwives. Individuals perceiving themselves to be in need of health care can directly access any of the above they deem appropriate.

In some respects this use of the term 'primary care' does most closely correspond to the model used by those involved in health service planning in its widest sense. However, we may reflect that currently in reality within the UK, professionals other than those described above (for example, district nurses, dietitians and physiotherapists or occupational therapists), whilst having a key role in the provision of community health services, can only be accessed via a referral system which is controlled by the medical profession.

To give two examples: first, although patients can contact community (i.e. district) nurses independently for initial advice (e.g. for incontinence), nurses cannot provide ongoing advice and support to patients unless they have a formal referral from a GP. Second, whilst a patient with back pain or suffering from the after-effects of a stroke or sports injury might benefit most from treatment by a physiotherapist, likewise within the NHS, the patient cannot directly access this professional but has to obtain a referral from a GP or other doctor.

Recent developments in health policy in England and Wales (DoH 1997), and in Scotland (SODoH 1997) show that in developing primary care, the government is seeking to retain elements of the primary care-led NHS, with its focus around the GP, but at the same time the new policies seek to broaden the base to include both other professionals and lay people and to spread the organisational structure and focus over a wider geographical area. Hence, at the time of writing, Primary Care Trusts, primary care groups in England and local health care co-ops in Scotland are to be the new organisational structures and they will comprise members from nursing and the local community as well as general practitioners from a group of practices.

Alongside the emergence of the term 'primary health care', with its associated assumption of the centrality of the GP, the term 'primary health-care team (PHCT)' also appeared, used to cover many of those working outside the hospital sector, but within the NHS. The term still had the implied assumption of the GP at its head but this use of the word 'team' implied a much more coherent relationship between these individuals than was generally the case. Indeed, it was rather unclear as to who was supposed to be in the 'team' – some took it to refer to the staff working in the immediate vicinity of the practice and employed by the GP, including practice nurses, the practice manager and reception and clerical staff. Other individuals and/or professions with key contributions to make within primary care, such as midwives, health visitors, district nurses and pharmacists, were sometimes included and sometimes not.

In general, these professionals were either employed by the local trust (as in the case of midwives, district nurses and health visitors) or were independent contractors (as in the case of pharmacists). Some, such as physiotherapists and occupational therapists, could only be accessed via the hospital system. Social services, who also have a key role in the management of individuals requiring ongoing support in the community, were rarely included.

We can see from the above that even the simple definition of terms poses problems in primary care and efforts to clarify some of these issues of definition and boundaries, and hence of responsibility and accountability, make for ongoing difficulties. The 'primary care team' approach can be seen at its best in the care of individual patients where professionals collaborate to provide the best package of care for that patient. Unfortunately, evidence collected by patients' support groups and charities all too frequently tell a tale of poor coordination and lack of joint planning and collaboration (Hunter & Wistow 1991). In addition, taking collaboration forward into the area of planning for the practice population as a whole, and involving professionals and local people in decision making, largely does not happen although the new structures may alter this.

This lack of coherence would appear to be more due to organisational and/or financial factors rather than being the fault of individual practitioners of any group. John Hasler, an eminent GP who played a significant part in the development of primary care as we know it today, commented in a monograph on the PHCT that the period following 1948 was difficult for GPs (Hasler 1994): 'It seemed as though family doctors had been left out in the cold whilst the hospitals with their technological and scientific advances forged ahead'.

Their contractual arrangements agreed in 1948 reinforced an individual approach and meant that if GPs spent significant money on premises, equipment or staff, this reduced their income. This resulted in few additional support staff being employed to ease the administrative load and build links across agencies. In addition, owing to the differing managerial arrangements for district nurses and health visitors, there was little if any contact between these nurses and GPs. In 1966, Lisbeth Hockey, from the Queen's Institute of District Nursing, published a survey of community nursing which identified these gaps (Hockey 1966). In particular, the survey found that doctors and nurses were unclear as to how they should work together.

At the time, the response to this was the development of GP attachment schemes, whereby district nurses and health visitors were 'attached' to GP practices and responsible for those registered populations rather than for geographical areas. This was not universally popular, either with the medical officers of health or with GPs. Nevertheless, despite initial resistance, by the early 1970s 75% of all district nurses and health visitors in England and Wales were attached to GP practices.

But the problems of lack of communication and poor collaboration continued and in 1986, potentially recreating, to some extent, the problems encountered prior to GP attachment schemes, the Cumberlege Report (DHSS 1986) took an alternative view, giving prominence to the nursing role within primary care. This report recommended the separation of nursing from general practice and that community nursing be organised in smaller units based in a defined geographical area or patch. The report concluded that:

- community nursing services should be planned, organised and delivered on a neighbourhood basis;
- there is scope for making better use of nursing skills;
- the effectiveness of the primary care team needs to be improved;
- there should be an integrated approach to the training of all nurses outside hospitals;
- consumer groups should have a stronger voice.

Possibly rendered cautious by memories of the lack of communication resulting from the previous organisation of community nursing services along geographical lines, the desire of GPs to retain nurses under their own control and to retain a GP practice focus for primary care, the government response to these recommendations as outlined in the White Paper *Promoting better health* (DHSS 1987) was to do nothing other than note the increase in community nurses since the late 1970s and refer to the wide variety of health authority staff employed. The White Paper alluded to the difference in employment status between nurses employed by the (then) health authorities and those working in general practice who were employed by the GPs themselves. It acknowledged the lack of training and career structure for practice nurses and recommended that these issues be addressed. But there was no attempt at this stage to reintroduce a geographically based nursing team structure or to integrate in any specific way the nursing services as provided through GP practices and those provided via the community services.

The next key influence was the new GP contract in 1990, which led to an increase in responsibilities within primary care and which in turn impacted on the role of nurses in primary care and in the community in general. White Papers at the time (*Working for patients* 1989, *Caring for people* 1989) further emphasised the role of the PHCT but continued to ignore the financial and organisational barriers to team working which existed in reality.

The White Paper *Working for patients* (DoH 1989a) finally introduced the reforms to the NHS and changed the role of primary care. It superseded *Promoting better health* (DHSS 1987) and provided the structure for the NHS during the 1990s. It introduced the concept of the so-called 'internal market' (Enthoven 1985), central to which was the theory that market forces were to be brought to bear within the NHS to promote economy and efficiency. In the reorganisation, some NHS organisations were given the role of 'purchasers' and others designated as 'providers'. Health authorities were key purchasers and NHS trust were providers, alongside some other health-care organisations in the private and voluntary sectors.

In primary care, most 'purchasing' was done by the health authorities, with GPs as providers, retaining their independent contractor status. However, with the intention of making purchasing decisions closer to local needs, a purchasing role was also given to some GPs, who became known as 'GP fundholders'. These GP practices, in addition to their role as normal GP service providers, held funds with which they could purchase certain kinds of services, including, latterly, community nursing. In this way, GPs were acting as 'proxy' for their patients but no requirement was placed on them to consult with patients or with other professionals working in the community. This gave increased power to GPs but vastly reduced the influence of community nurses, in particular that of health visitors, whose public health role had never been adequately understood by GPs.

However, the most recent White Papers (DoH 1997, SoDoh 1997), dealing with the restructuring of the NHS to further develop the primary care-led NHS, offers some redress and increases the potential for nurses to take a greater role in the provision of community health services. It is intended that nurses will have a greater say within primary care groups (PCGs) or local health care co-ops (LHCCs) and legislation has paved the way for the introduction of pilot schemes to promote the development of nurse-led services. But only time will tell whether the nursing profession is able to shift the focus from the medically dominated model to a more holistic and participative model of health care.

NURSES IN PRIMARY CARE

It will be useful at this stage to touch in more detail on how nursing roles are configured within primary care. Within the accepted model of GP-centred primary care, nurses generally come into three main categories, although other groups of nurses work in community settings outside the main structures of primary care.

Working from the practice outwards, the first category identified is that of practice nurses, employed by the GP to work with patients of that practice. Practice nurses have greatly increased in number since the introduction of the new GP contract (Atkin et al 1993). Although now a professional group by virtue of their numbers and the change in role of GP practices, there is still no formal educational preparation for becoming a practice nurse other than basic nurse training, nor are they a professional group recognised by statute as are health visitors and district nurses. GPs, as independent contractors and employers, largely control the extent to which practice nurses can access appropriate training and education. As a result, the educational provision for these nurses is patchy and task focused and GPs remain reluctant to release them or to pay for them to undertake longer, university-based, educational programmes which they perceive to be of little immediate relevance to the clinical needs of their patients. Practice nurses also only work with patients of an individual practice and this poses a considerable barrier to them working with communities as a whole. In areas of work such as health promotion (e.g. teenage sexual health), where it may be necessary to work across a number of agencies to be effective, this limitation is extremely problematic.

A second category is that of community nurses (formerly known as 'district nurses'). These nurses are usually employed by a local NHS trust and provide 'hands-on' nursing care to patients in their homes. District nursing grew out of home nursing services provided by local authorities and did not become part of the NHS as such until 1974. It was only as recently as 1968 (Baly et al 1987) that the professional qualification of district nurse was officially recognised, but gradually education for district nurses has been included in the portfolio offered by university departments of nursing. Currently, home nursing services are provided by a team of district or community nurses, not all of whom will have the professional qualification. However, community nursing teams are always led by trained community nurses who undertake the nursing assessments and then delegate the provision of care to an appropriately skilled individual, whilst retaining overall responsibility for care provided.

District or community nurses are now almost always attached to one or more GP practices and frequently based within practice premises, leading to generally improved communication regarding the care of individual patients. However, the employing authority to whom they are accountable is still usually the NHS trust provider, who has overall responsibility for nursing policy, and it is still the case that district nurses working at local level are hardly ever included in the process of planning care for the whole practice population. They frequently have few links with their professional colleagues, the practice nurses, and in this way, opportunities working collaboratively, such as in the care of elderly patients or those who have chronically disabling conditions, are lost (Audit Commission 1992).

A third category is that of the health visitor or public health nurse. This group is also employed by local NHS trusts and now usually has an attachment to one or more GP practices. Health visitors were also originally employed by local authorities and their work derived from a perceived public health need to address the health of mothers and young children. They have been the most highly trained of nurses working in the community, until recently being the only nurses who could lay claim to a university education. This was a broad-based qualification theoretically enabling them to work with people 'from cradle to grave' but in reality, most retain a role which largely concerns mothers and young children. Even within this narrow focus, however, the role of the health visitor is even more constrained by the medical model, which focuses on individuals and generally does not encompass the wider community.

In the care of young children, health visitors need to work with a great range of community agencies – nurseries, childminders and social services, to name but a few – and health visitors themselves see their role as going beyond the achievement of immunisation targets (a key area and remuneration target for GPs), however important these may be. However, targets are easy to measure, unlike the outcomes for 'softer' areas such as the development of support for new mothers, and within the new 'evidence-based' NHS, it has proved difficult to establish a strong evidence base for the work of health visitors. Working with families may extend over many years and outcomes are difficult to measure appropriately. This lack of evidence of effectiveness has led to the further marginalisation of health visitors who find themselves perceived as expensive professionals whose tasks might be undertaken by less expensive, more easily controlled, practice nurses. The current government's concern with broader public health issues, together with the introduction of PCGs with a community focus, may provide the health visitors with an ideal opportunity to reinvent themselves and their role with the wider community.

There is an emerging fourth category of nurses within GP-led primary care, which is that of 'nurse practitioner'. This is a new and developing role where nurses, usually but not always, employed by a GP, have undertaken further education and training to equip them to both diagnose and treat a wider range of illness. Such nurses work autonomously and despite not being able to actually write their own prescriptions, they carry their own caseload and refer to GPs or other health professionals as they deem appropriate. Their work has been described as 'doctor substitution' rather than nursing, although the nurse practitioners themselves deny this and argue that their nursing background enables them to work more holistically and beyond the medical model. There are now some examples of primary care pilots (not yet fully evaluated) which are based around a nurse practitioner model and some GP practices employ nurse practitioners, but so far the qualification is not recognised in law.

However, if the model of primary care is widened to include community services outside GP practices, we immediately find a whole range of other categories of nurses working within primary and community care settings. These groups include community and/or independent midwives, who may be GP attached but are in law autonomous practitioners; community psychiatric nurses, who are employed by mental health NHS trusts and whose role is largely with people who have long-term and chronic serious mental health problems; and nurses working with people with learning difficulties in the community. Other groups also exist, such as Macmillan nurses, who are funded to work with patients with cancer in the community (usually those who are terminally ill), and school nurses, whose role is largely perceived to be dealing with immunisation programmes and minor health problems such as head lice, despite potentially having a role in other areas such as adolescent and sexual health through having access to an otherwise rather inaccessible population group.

Although space does not permit us to look in depth at the work of these latter groups, considering community and primary care nursing in this way provides immediate insight into the limitations of a GP practice-focused model of primary care and it will be helpful at this stage to explore possible different approaches and ways of integrating a wider public health model within existing ways of working.

BEYOND A MEDICAL MODEL OF PRIMARY CARE

Our exploration above of the definitions of primary care, description of its historical development and organisational structure, together with the identification of current nursing roles within it, has highlighted the narrowness of the current medical model and the potential for nursing to expand the model to include a public health perspective. What might a new model look like?

As already noted, a particular model of 'primary care' occurs where the term is used as a form of shorthand for 'primary medical care' (Macdonald 1992, Pratt 1995), i.e. primary care operating through medical practice and the GP. This model concentrates on illness and medically defined solutions to health needs. It emerges clearly in the definition provided by the Royal College of General Practitioners (RCGP 1972) which uses the term 'primary care' as almost synonymous with 'general practice'.

...personal, primary and continuing medical care to individuals and families ... (The doctor) will intervene educationally, preventatively and therapeutically to promote his (sic) patient's health.

An expanded model of primary health care can be found within the WHO Health for All strategy which defined primary health care as:

...essential health care based on practical, scientifically sound and socially acceptable methods and technology made universally available to individuals and families in the community through their full participation.

Primary care supporting this latter model could be referred to as 'the public health model of primary care', where communities are involved alongside a range of professionals in the planning and delivery of local health services.

Such a model is reflected in current projects described in a study undertaken by the Public Health Alliance (Peckham et al 1996) and in community-oriented primary care (COPC) developed in the USA which combines the care of individuals and families in the community (Abramson 1984). This model emphasises aspects which are wider than the medical model and explicitly acknowledges the significant contribution of broader social issues such as housing, transport, nutrition and education, to health and well-being. The WHO Health for All strategy also attaches importance to the principles of intersectoral working, the diminution of professional hierarchies, the pursuit of equity and the participation of the community.

Taking these ideas further, the view of people as having both the right and the duty to participate in the planning and delivery of their own health care has been more recently reinterpreted to define three sets of activity (WHO 1991). These are:

- 'a contribution by people to their own health and health care;
- the development of organisational structures that are needed for participation to be effective;
- the empowerment of patients and their organisations and advocates so that their voice is heard, not assumed.'

In this context it is interesting to contrast the model of primary care prevalent in the UK with the model described above. Health service policy during the 1980s, following the political leaning of the time, promoted an approach which was individualistic rather than social. Indeed, the report of the NHS review in the 1980s, *Promoting better health* (DoH 1987), which heralded the start of the subsequent NHS reforms, largely ignored community approaches and focused specifically on the organisation and delivery of professional services and on individual responsibility. For example, in the section on preventable disease (DoH 1987, pp. 2–3, para. 1.1) it is noted:

Much of this distress and suffering could be avoided if more members of the public took greater responsibility for looking after their own health. The Government fully acknowledges its responsibility for raising individuals' awareness of the ways in which they can continue to take steps to maintain good health.

However, this emphasis on individual responsibility failed to deliver the hoped-for improvements and more recent changes, in the face of increasing inequalities in health (e.g. Wilkinson 1996), have led to UK health initiatives such as PCGs and LHCCs, which encourage 'bottom-up' participative approaches, and a movement towards a public health approach.

DEFINING PUBLIC HEALTH

But if we have spent time considering definitions and models of primary care, what of public health, the wider dimension we have talked about? The literature on public health offers a range of definitions, from a pure epidemiological/communicable disease approach to something which is more active and about changing health (Harris 1995).

For example, on the one hand, definitions of public health can be drawn very narrowly around hygiene or epidemic disease control with a focus on population approaches rather than on individuals and as a discipline, public health medicine has used mainly epidemiological approaches identifying particular health risks. For example, in prevention of coronary heart disease, a traditional public health approach would be to determine those most at risk and focus prevention programmes on individual risk factor reduction for this population.

On the other hand, definitions of public health can be broadened to encompass social resources and all forms of health care. The Acheson Report (DHSS 1988) adopted a definition of public health based on one developed by the World Health Authority in 1952, namely: '...the science and art of preventing disease, prolonging life and promoting health through organised efforts of society'.

One element of the debate has been the distinction between public health as a *resource* and public health as a *service*. This debate is at the heart of many current discussions about the role of public health including public health nursing, health promotion and environmental health. But a complicating feature is that clearly many of the activities of health promotion work and public health nursing, in particular health visitors, represent a public health approach at both individual reactive (service) and population preventive (resource) levels.

In the UK, the lay view of public health has been that of local authorities taking the lead role in terms of responsibility for issues such as sanitation, provision of housing, environmental issues and social welfare measures. The professional view (particularly in recent years) has been of public health as an academic discipline, researching and identifying patterns of diseases and mechanisms for their control.

We saw earlier that community health services and the public health role in terms of the management of disease were originally developed within local authorities and were only taken over by the NHS in 1974.

Although this move was made in order to facilitate the coordinated delivery of community health services, the removal of community health services from local authorities severed the link between social care, housing and environment. This had the effect of moving the focus of public health as a service for social and environmental care to the biomedical and epidemiological model.

However, with the advent of the Healthy Cities initiative (Ashton 1986) and the Health for All programme (Faculty of Community Medicine 1972), many local authorities were able to reclaim a 'public health role' and recent health policy has shown signs of reinventing a broader public health perspective and the need for collaboration. For example, there has been increasing recognition of the links between housing and ill health and poverty and of socioeconomic issues relating to variations in health (Ashton & Seymour 1998).

We have noted that *The health of the nation* (1991) (DoH 1991) and also *Promoting better health* (DHSS 1987) concentrated primarily on individuals' responsibility for their own health, particularly in avoiding unhealthy lifestyles. The professional role was identified as solely that of education and advice. This ignored the findings of previous reports on structural influences on health, and in particular the Black Report (1980) and the Whitehead publication (1988) on inequality and health. But following the change in government in 1997, health inequalities have returned to the forefront and have been made a priority for both health and local authorities. Health inequalities have been made an overarching priority in the most recent health White Papers (DoH 1999, SODoH 1999). It will be important for health professionals, including most particularly community and primary care nurses, to grasp the possibilities that this new emphasis will offer.

THE NEW PUBLIC HEALTH

Ashton & Seymour (1988) have defined the new public health as:

...an approach which brings together environmental change and personal preventive measures with appropriate therapeutic interventions [but which] goes beyond an understanding of human biology and recognizes the importance of those social aspects of health problems which are caused by life-styles.

The new public health was given legitimacy through the above-mentioned WHO Health for All policy which had three main objectives:

1. promotion of lifestyles conducive to health;
2. prevention of preventable conditions;
3. rehabilitation and health services.

These objectives were derived from a range of goals or targets developed for each WHO region in 1985 and the UK is signatory to the European targets (WHO 1985). A key aim of the European programme is to shift the emphasis away from a narrow medical view by:

- promoting self-care;
- integration of medical care with other related activities such as education and recreation;
- environmental improvements and social welfare (intersectoral action);
- integrating the promotion of good health with preventive medicine, treatment and rehabilitation;
- meeting the needs of underserved groups;
- community participation.

Health promotion is a key element of the new public health approach and how it might be operationalised is enshrined in the later Ottawa charter (WHO 1986) which stated that health promotion should:

- be based on the active involvement of the population;
- direct action on the causes of ill health;
- combine a range of approaches aimed at improving health;
- recognise the important role of all health workers.

Throughout all this, we can identify key elements to a public health approach. These are:

- equity (the focus on underserved groups, improving health for all),
- collaboration (the need to work intersectorally),
- participation (the need to involve the public in improving their health), and
- strengthening community action.

Equity in the National Health Service

As Wilkinson (1996) has noted, a commitment to equity is fundamental to the achievement of improved health and it is implicit within the principles of the new public health as outlined above. But it is not always clear what this might mean or how primary care professionals can integrate this commitment into their working practice. One way of doing this is to ensure that people can play an active part in the planning and delivery of services and it is possible for primary care professionals to actively encourage participation and community involvement in their practice.

If carried out at a community level, this is a more helpful approach to equity which draws on participation and advocacy in order to include people in the decisions surrounding health and health care. Within primary care, it means a greater commitment to a wider approach than care of the individuals of a practice population and will include a need to develop policies which empower professionals who may act as advocates for their patients or clients, as well as mechanisms to facilitate the involvement of service users themselves. Finally, and importantly, it will require a structure of accountability at a local level. Within public health, this will mean closer links with local authorities and the re-emphasising of the importance of housing, transport, environment and education as well as the provision of clinical health services and the management of specific diseases.

Moving towards a public health model of primary care

From an exploration of the definitions of primary care and public health and a discussion of the principles of equity as described above, it is possible to identify some common ground between primary health care and public health. Key elements of this overlap relate to a community/population focus, health prevention/promotion and community participation. All raise issues of equity and the need to collaborate with other agencies and thus we can see that the same three pillars – equity, collaboration and participation – provide the common threads to both public health and primary health care.

It is also clear that primary health-care professionals, and GPs in particular, need to be drawn into wider public health debates about equity, appropriateness and effectiveness of services. This requires an awareness of how local people perceive existing services and a knowledge of local needs, not just those demanded by specific patients in the surgery but wider needs of local communities. We need to draw on a much broader definition of primary health care which, as Macdonald (1992) has argued, should include not only health-care professionals but also other primary care workers, such as environmental health, teachers and social workers and input from communities.

The overlap can also be seen to include epidemiological work, communicable disease control and support relating to clinical decision making. Thus, the range of activity described by health authority directors of public health (Peckham et al 1996) must be incorporated into any public health model of primary health care alongside a range of other approaches such as Healthy City and Health for All activities, community health projects, health and housing projects and health promotion work in schools.

Thus it is possible to view public health and primary health care as overlapping circles (Fig. 11.1). The circles representing primary health care and public health overlap where both interact with a third circle representing the community to promote collaboration and participation and it is the community which is touched by both public health and primary care.

Primary health care, public health and participation

But what do we mean by participation and community involvement?

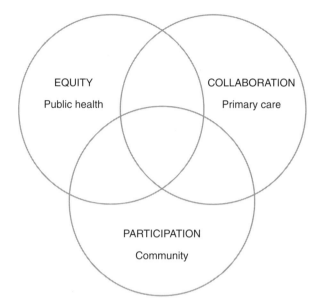

Fig. 11.1   A model of a public health approach to primary care.

Public involvement in planning and decision making has been largely absent in the traditional biomedical model in both public health and primary care. In the initial stages of the NHS, there was little or no attempt to involve the public in the planning or delivery of health care, outside the use of volunteers in hospitals and the presence of community representatives on public bodies such as health boards and family practitioner committees. In 1974, community health councils were introduced, with statutory rights to information and entry to health authority premises, but their role was severely weakened following the NHS reforms of 1990. At this time CHCs were given rights in relation to health authorities but not to NHS trusts, which were deemed independent provider organisations. Subsequently, patients were given what were, in fact, largely illusory consumer rights through the 'patients' charters' which NHS organisations were required to produce but which emphasised the 'consumer' element, rather than a basic human right.

Within primary care, particularly during the 1970s and early 1980s, there was a movement towards 'patient participation' and some practices developed patient groups. Some of these groups came to play an active part in the delivery of services, particularly in relation to the care of elderly people registered with the practice. Some continue to do so. But they have only existed with the consent of the participating GPs, they have played

Table 11.1 A continuum of public involvement demonstrating progress towards a public health model of primary care

Primary health care activity	Level	Public health activity
Reactive medical practive focused on the sick individual	Weak	Evidence-based medicine, tertiary prevention
Population (GP list)-focused care, some proactive medicine but still individual based	Intermediate	Population data from GP system, mainly quantitative in nature, practice profiles, concern with communicable and chronic diseases
Multiprofessional (intrasectoral) team work, proactive with focus on prevention, community-orientated primary care	Strong	Health promotion, local health needs assessment. Rehabilitation processes linked with local community resources. Epidemiological data from public health depts for whole area, not just practice
Multiprofessional (intersectoral), community based, proactive (including concern for addressing needs of disadvantaged groups), mechanisms for community involvement	Synthesis	Participative and collaborative needs assessment and health promotion (e.g. PRA), active partnerships with community health groups Drawing on wider public health skills as well as community resources

little or no part in either planning services or providing advocates for patients in the practice and they have no statutory rights.

Active involvement of the local community to promote health within primary care would therefore be an essential component of a public health model of primary care. As well as the conceptual model given in Figure 11.1, this can be demonstrated as a continuum of activity, as in Table 11.1 where the element of public participation is shown as progressing from weak (i.e. the traditional model focusing on the sick individual) through to a model which demonstrates a synthesis of shared planning and implementation between individuals, health professionals and the community.

There are two further specific points that need to be addressed which relate to the issue of participation. The first is that participation operates at both an individual and collective level but individual empowerment and involvement are often only expressible and achieved through collective action. The second is that there are different degrees or levels of participation. These have been described elsewhere by Arnstein (1969) as a ladder of progression from tokenistic participation and relative powerlessness to full democratic participation.

In health care we can see how these levels might work in action from token consultation processes with no proper representation from or feedback to the community or real power to influence events (the most usual level of local involvement currently), through to situations where people have a right to be represented, can choose their representatives, have the power to veto decisions with which they disagree and also to contribute to the delivery of decisions made.

TOWARDS A PUBLIC HEALTH MODEL OF PRIMARY CARE: AN EXAMPLE IN PRACTICE

A detailed example of how this can work in practice is given below. The example is hypothetical but is drawn from similar case studies identified during a research project into public health and primary care. Only one in-depth example is given, to enable us to see how the same problem can be tackled either at a superficial level using an approach based on the medical model or via a community-based approach incorporating a wide range of individuals and agencies. Once you get a feel for the wider approach, it is easy to look for examples from other areas such as community nursing, care of the elderly and mental health.

The example is given as a vignette and then demonstrates four levels of involvement, which equate to the four levels shown in Table 11.1. With each level there is movement towards a public health approach, with an increase in the participation of patients and the community, a drawing together of public health and primary care approaches and the involvement of a wider range of professionals and agencies.

Vignette

A health visitor has on her caseload in a deprived area a family with four children aged 12, 10, 6 and 3. Two of the children, the eldest and the 3-year-old, have asthma which is poorly controlled. The eldest child is frequently absent from school, particularly when it is 'games' as he finds it difficult to participate. Both parents smoke. The 10-year-old has also been caught smoking in the playground of the primary school. Father works as casual labourer when there is building work around. He is usually out during the day.

Level 1 response – reactive medical practice focused on the sick individual

Health visitor visits frequently and advises mother on care of 3-year-old. Advises her to take child to GP to improve asthma care and suggests older children go as well. Is sympathetic, but advises mother she should stop smoking if possible.

Mother takes children to GP, who also advises her to stop smoking and prescribes more inhalers for the children. He tells the eldest child that he must take his 'preventers' for his asthma. He refers the family to the asthma clinic with the practice nurse.

Practice nurse teaches both children (and mother) how to use inhaler and also advises mother to stop smoking. They are told to come back if there are continuing problems, which they do, repeatedly.

Health visitor continues to visit and support.

Comment

The above reflects what is probably the most common response to such a problem. The professionals are sympathetic and have read all the literature about what medication is appropriate. They are aware of the links between smoking and ill health. They work conscientiously within their perceived remit. They are often not very successful in helping the patients because their work is mainly composed of 'telling' the patients what to do and what is best for them. They tend to develop a worldview of patients as 'non-compliant'.

The health visitor sees her role as working with preschool children and mother and she feels she has too heavy a caseload to do any more.

There are no regular team meetings between health visitor and the GP practice team, although discussions take place around individual cases.

Level 2 response – population focused, some proactive medicine, but still individual based

Actions take place as at level 1.

After seeing the family, it occurs to the GP that there seem to be quite a lot of children in the practice with asthma and quite a lot of adults who smoke. He discusses this with the practice nurse and the practice manager and they do a search on the list which indicates that this is indeed the case. He contacts the pharmaceutical representative and asks for a supply of leaflets for childhood asthma and smoking cessation.

The practice nurse makes sure that she gives the leaflets to the family and others where appropriate.

The GP and practice nurse audit their asthma clinic regularly and notice that patients still don't like using the preventers and that most of the adults continue to smoke. They are frustrated at their apparent inability to get through to patients, who continue to turn up with badly controlled asthma and a need for sick notes from school. They think the health visitor should be able to advise the family on smoking, because 'health visitors do health promotion'.

The health visitor continues to visit as before. She is sympathetic and says she has a lot of families where asthma is a problem. She hasn't done any specialist training in asthma or smoking prevention, so she is unable to advise the family with regard to either the children's asthma or the parents' smoking. Anyway, she sees it as the role of the GP and practice nurse to tackle the patients about smoking cessation because 'they get paid for health promotion'.

Comments

What we see here is an increasing awareness within the immediate primary care team that there is a problem which needs to be dealt with.

The good medical care is continuing, with the concerned GP interested enough to look at the numbers of patients on his list with asthma and who smoke. He may also be interested enough to look at the prescribing costs for patients with asthma and the number of times such patients attend. He continues to make sure that he is up to date with clinical treatment and sends his nurse on courses.

The clinic is very efficient but neither nurse or GP feels that it is very effective, although they don't see themselves as having the time to do anything else.

The practice nurse does not see it as her role to take the initiative. Neither she nor the GP talks to the health visitor, so neither side is aware of what the other can or cannot do. Nobody has talked to anyone in the community at all.

The health visitor doesn't see what else she can do, as the GP runs the asthma clinic. She waits for the doctor to do something.

Level 3 response – multiprofessional, intersectoral teamwork, proactive, with focus on prevention: community-orientated primary care

The good basic care continues, but the health visitor decides that something should be done with all these children with asthma.

She audits her own caseload and does a brief summary of the problem for her manager. She talks to the mothers and all agree that having children with asthma is very problematic – parents get very tired and stressed. They decide to ask the doctor to one of their mothers' discussion groups and get him to talk to them about it.

The doctor talks to the mothers and the health visitor talks to the practice nurse. The practice nurse agrees to teach the health visitor about asthma and the use of inhalers. The health visitor suggests that she might come to the clinic and help in the discussion with the mothers. They arrange for a volunteer to look after the children in the clinic whilst they talk with the mothers. During this discussion, the subject of smoking comes up and several of the women say that they would like to give up but find it hard to do it on their own. A 'stop smoking' group is suggested and one of the mothers says they could meet in her house if the health visitor can help them.

The health visitor, GP and practice nurse feel more encouraged with all of this and agree to help to follow up these initiatives and to have regular meetings and review how they are getting on.

Comments

The practice team are beginning to understand that it may look like more work to meet and discuss with others but they feel, and are, more effective.

The GP is glad he doesn't have to take the initiative. The practice nurse finds the health visitor helpful and she will visit patients who don't turn up to the clinic. The health visitor feels more confident because she understands more of the clinical side. The families feel more supported and are more confident to address their own health issues. They understand more about the medicines they are asked to take and don't get so worried and tired. They are more aware of asthma and respiratory problems and concerned about the traffic fumes. They talk to other parents in the playground and become aware of people who have similar problems who go to other doctors.

Level 4 response – multiprofessional, intersectoral, community based, proactive

The medical care continues. The asthma clinic continues to run.

The parents ask the health visitor to talk to the parents' evening at the primary school and she is then asked to talk to the secondary school. In so doing, she meets the school nurse and they discuss the problem. The school nurse keeps all the inhalers in a cupboard and children have to ask for them because of the 'dangers of drugs', according to the headmaster. She says that a lot of the children with asthma don't do PE.

The parents decide to have an open evening at the school and the health visitor helps by going to the local health promotion department for information and posters on smoking cessation. The HP department offer help in getting a no-smoking policy adopted in the school which is accepted.

As part of the open evening, the public health department from the local health authority is asked to come and talk about asthma in the local community. They also ask the environmental health department in the local authority for information about traffic pollution.

The local chemist, who has a child at the school, runs a window display and special promotion on smoking cessation.

All the local GPs help the school carry out a policy of children keeping their inhalers with them and give a lunchtime talk to the PE staff about asthma and exercise. It is suggested to have a swimming club in the local baths particularly for children with asthma … and so on and so on.

Comments

By this level, a large range of agencies, professionals and individuals are getting in on the act. It is likely that all of this will make a significant impact on a range of problems associated with the health of the community. People are involved and proactive and using the professionals for advice and support. By getting the problem away from individuals and out into the wider community, it is possible to achieve much more, without greatly, if at all, increasing the need for professional resources. However, a willingness to collaborate and a willingness to 'power share' are essential components of such an approach. The key words for effectiveness here are: **equity, collaboration and participation**.

CONCLUSION

The development of primary health care and its role in the overall promotion of health is a vital component of a strategy to improve health. However, if it is to be effective in doing this, as opposed to confining activity to the commissioning of secondary services, then a broad collaborative approach, with opportunities for the community to participate, will be essential. In particular, the role of nurses and health visitors needs to become more visible than it currently is within the framework of primary care. If the principles which appear to underpin the development of the new primary care groups can be actively incorporated into practice alongside clear lines of accountability and the inclusion of patients in the decision-making process, then a public health model of primary care should assist in achieving real health gain.

REFERENCES

Abel-Smith B 1960 A history of the nursing profession. Heinemann, London
Abramson J H 1984 Application of epidemiology in community orientated primary care. Public Health Report 99(5): 437–442
Arnstein S 1969 A ladder of citizen participation. Journal of the American Institute of Planners 35: 216–224
Ashton J 1986 Healthy cities. Health Promotion 1(2): 319–324
Ashton J, Seymour H 1988 The new public health: the Liverpool experience. Open University Press, Milton Keynes
Atkin K, Lunt N, Parker G, Hirst M 1993 Nurses count – a national census of practice nurses. Social Policy Research Unit, University of York
Audit Commission 1992 Homeward bound: a new course for community health. HMSO, London
Baly M, Robottom B, Clark J 1987 District nursing. Heinemann, London
Black D (Chair) 1980 Inequalities in health. Report of a research working group. HMSO, London
DHSS 1986 Neighbourhood nursing – a focus of care (the Cumberlege Report). HMSO, London
DHSS 1987 Promoting better health – the government's programme for improving primary health care. HMSO, London
DHSS 1988 Report of the public health in England – the Acheson report. HMSO, London
DoH 1989a Working for patients. HMSO, London
DoH 1989b Caring for people. HMSO, London
DOH 1991 The health of the nation – a consultative document. HMSO, London
DoH 1997 The new NHS: modern, dependable. HMSO, London
DoH 1998 Our healthier nation. HMSO London
Enthoven A 1985 Reflections on the management of the National Health Service. Nuffield Provincial Hospitals Trust, London
Faculty of Community Medicine 1972 Health for all by the year 2000 – charter for action. Faculty of Community Medicine, London

Gamble E 1974 Primary care.

Harris S 1995 In: Laughlin S, Black D (eds). Poverty and health: tools for change; ideas, analysis, information, action. Public Health Alliance, Birmingham

Hasler J C 1994 The primary health care team. John Fry Trust Fellowship Monograph. Royal Society of Medicine, London

Hockey L 1966 Feeling the pulse. Queen's Institute of District Nursing, London

Hunter D J, Wistow G 1991 Elderly people's integrated care system (EPICS): an organisational, policy and practice review. Nuffield Institute reports no. 3. Nuffield Institute for Health Services Studies, University of Leeds, Leeds

Klein R 1989 The politics of the National Health Service, 2nd edn. Longman, Harlow

Macdonald J 1992 Primary health care: medicine in its place. Earthscan, London

Peckham S, Macdonald J, Taylor P 1996 Primary care and public health – project report phase 1. Public Health Alliance, Birmingham

Pratt J 1995 practitioners and practices: a conflict of values? Radcliffe Medical Press, Oxford

RCGP 1972 The future general practitioner: learning and teaching. Royal College of General Practitioners, London

SODoH 1997 Designed to care. HMSO, Edinburgh

SODoH 1999 Towards a healthier Scotland. Stationery Office, Edinburgh

Webster C 1993 Speaking out for the public's health. Papers from a conference on Public Health Advocacy. Public Health Alliance, Birmingham

Whitehead M 1988 The health divide. In Black D (Ed) Inequalities in health. Penguin, Harmondsworth

WHO 1985 Targets for all – targets in support of the European Regional Strategy for Health for All. WHO, Copenhagen

WHO 1986 Ottawa charter for health promotion. An international conference on health promotion. WHO, Copenhagen

WHO 1991 Community involvement in health development – report of a WHO study group. WHO technical report series no. 809. World Health Organisation, Geneva

Wilkinson R 1996 Unhealthy societies: the afflictions of inequality. Routledge, London

Policy issues in public health

12

Health outcome measurement

Di Douglas   Grace Lindsay

INTRODUCTION

This chapter will examine the concept of 'outcome' as it is used in modern health-care systems. A definition of the term 'outcome' and a summary of the main components will be provided together with an overview of some of the commonly associated terminology. Issues relating to timing of outcome assessment, attribution of results to care delivered, sensitivity, reliability and validity will be considered. The development of tools to measure the impact of health-care interventions will be described from a conceptual and technical perspective and, with use of examples, their applicability in the evaluation of health outcome will be discussed. Targets for health improvement outlined in recent government documents will be reviewed and the recommended health outcomes that should be monitored, at a population level, to assess progress in health improvement.

HEALTH OUTCOME MEASUREMENT: HISTORICAL PERSPECTIVE

The measurement of health outcomes can be traced back to the works of Florence Nightingale (Nightingale 1859) who is said to have used the three outcome measures of 'alive', 'dead' or 'relieved' to evaluate patient care. The use of survival and mortality statistics remains the cornerstone of health outcome assessment at a population level today. The term 'relieved' suggested that some assessment had been made in relation to improvement in the presenting condition, perhaps in changes in symptoms or treatments required to allow patients to live independently of health-care interventions. It is in this area that most advancement has taken place over the last 20 years in terms of identifying a framework through which assessment tools can be developed. The development of measurement tools to assess degree of change in different dimensions of health has provided a large number of potentially useful instruments for use in health outcome assessment.

HEALTH OUTCOME MEASUREMENT WITHIN QUALITY HEALTH CARE

A framework consisting of the three major components, namely structure, process and outcome, has been used to describe key areas of health care through which quality of health care may be evaluated (Donabedian 1980). This framework refers to the following areas of health care.

- *Structure* – relating to such factors as geographical setting, health-care facilities and resources.
- *Process* – describes the way health care is delivered such as the components of different care procedures, the manner in which they are carried out and the individual practitioners involved.
- *Outcome* – assesses the change in health status as a result of the health-care intervention. This may be based on a single dimension such as pain relief or on more global terms such as all-cause mortality.

Outcome assessment can therefore be regarded as one of the dimensions used in evaluation of quality of health care provision. Outcome assessment has been defined as the end result of medical care in terms of what happened to the patient and may be palliation, control of illness, cure or rehabilitation (Lohr 1988). The principal uses of outcome assessment have been described as the:

provision of a description of the impact of care ... the generation of information for reliable clinical decision making ... and the evaluation of the effectiveness of care under defined circumstances. (Davis et al 1994)

Outcome measures have been used to observe changes over time following a particular intervention and to test causality in the relationship between an intervention and a defined outcome (Hutchinson et al 1996).

OUTCOME TERMINOLOGY

Throughout the literature, numerous terms have been used in an attempt to encapsulate and convey the meaning of the term 'outcome' and its application within the context of health care. In an attempt to clarify and identify some common meanings within the different terms used, an analysis of these terms has been undertaken and conceptual themes extracted (Shanks & Frater 1993). These themes represent the possible components of outcomes described in the literature and provide some insights into the way the terminology associated with outcomes has been applied.

Four interlinking and recurrent themes have been drawn from the literature and one, several or all of these may be implied in any definition or application of outcome assessment. These themes are:

1. outcomes refer to the results of care;
2. outcomes reflect a change in one or more dimensions of 'health';
3. outcomes are attributed to interventions;
4. outcomes are predetermined, expected and/or anticipated.

Outcome as 'results' of care

There is general consensus in the published literature that an 'outcome' can be considered to be a result, or accumulation of results, of care (Brook et al 1976, Del Bueno 1993, Clark 1983, Jennings 1991). While some authors such as Donabedian (1969), Long et al (1993) and Fries (1983) have defined an 'outcome' as the result(s) of care, others have considered it as the end result(s) of care (Norman & Redfern 1993). Two interrelated points should be considered. First, when does the end result of care occur? The outcome of an intervention, particularly in preventive health care, may not be recognisable for several years, whereas some treatments may produce immediate results. Second, what is the most appropriate, feasible and practical time to measure the outcome? The effect of some interventions may be measured at various time points. The idea of multiple assessment has been suggested by Lohr (1988) who categorised time points for outcome assessment as 'short term, long term, or anything in between'. The most appropriate time point for measurement will, however, be determined by the nature of the intervention, the anticipated desired outcome and the type of measurement tool employed. The nature of the interventions may range from very short-term care delivery, for instance the administration of GTN to relieve symptoms of myocardial ischaemia, expected to act within a period of 10–15 minutes, to a much longer term assessment required to assess the impact of smoking cessation on general health and well-being. For this, a relevant time frame may be a period of months and even years.

Outcome as a measure of change in one or several dimensions of health status

Health-care interventions are directed toward and influence numerous aspects of health status. An individual's response(s) to interventions affects different aspects of health status (e.g. psychological or functional status). The results of health-care interventions therefore can be examined from a number of perspectives. The term 'health status' in this context has been used broadly and refers to a set of wide-ranging concepts extending from knowledge, attitude and satisfaction to physical, social and psychological functioning. Health status, according to Marek (1989), may include the dimensions of psychological, physical, behavioural, spiritual and functional well-being.

Health care is a multidimensional activity provided in a variety of situations, by many individuals, with numerous environmental, social, physical and organisational variables influencing the outcome. Yet, outcomes are frequently viewed in relation to a particular dimension of health care such as from the perspective of a specific provider of care or the symptomatic effect of an intervention to relieve pain. However, as Waters (1986) argues, it is often difficult to ascertain which interventions are responsible for a specific outcome and whether it is realistic to expect that health outcome can ever be attributable solely to nursing activities (Van Maanen 1981, Bond & Thomas 1992). Similarly, some factors may be independent of the care intervention, although they have an impact on it. The ability of a client to get better or otherwise, for instance, may be as a result of inherent capabilities or a decline in health status might occur despite nursing interventions (Barriball & MacKenzie 1993). This notion has been supported by Bloch (1975) and Bond (1992) who assert that patients' knowledge, feelings, behaviour and health state are influenced by many factors apart from community services in relation to health promotion. In addition, the longer the period of time between the intervention and the outcome assessment, the weaker the connection between outcomes and processes of care because of the possible influence of many extraneous factors.

Outcome attributable to an intervention

Donabedian (1980) defined health outcome as 'a change in a patient's current and future health status that can be attributed to antecedent care'. This definition incorporated the notion that only the endpoint of the intervention that can be directly attributed to the process of intervention has meaning and not all changes that may occur. The importance of establishing attribution, or care provider effects as it is termed by Jennings (1991), is echoed by many authors (Donabedian 1966, 1969, 1989, Marek 1989, Bloch 1975). 'Attribution' is concerned with linking or relating structural or procedural interventions directly with outcome. This may be strong enough to be considered as a 'cause and effect' relationship. In this instance, the outcome (e.g. change in health status) occurred as a direct effect of the structure or process of care (Burback & Quarry 1991). The strongest association from a statistical point of view is that of a 'cause and effect' relationship. However, in reality, such a relationship between structure, process and outcome remains difficult to prove for a particular intervention (Clark 1983, Shanks & Frater 1993). There is, for example, a large body of evidence that supports the causal relationship of smoking to lung cancer but many other interventions or lifestyle behaviours have a much weaker association with health-care outcome (Doll et al 1994).

Outcomes that are predetermined, expected and/or anticipated

Norman & Redfern (1993) state that 'An outcome refers to the expected changes in predetermined factors such as the patient's behaviour, health status or knowledge following the completion of nursing care'. Outcomes may be aspects of care that result in no ill effect or no changes, such as the absence of pressure sores or wound infections, as well as those that do happen, e.g. the impact of drugs on the cardiovascular system.

It is generally accepted within the area of health-care provision that responses to interventions are predetermined, expected or anticipated. On the whole, it would be unreasonable for a treatment, for example, to be administered if the result of this intervention had never been considered. In some instances, however, the range of expected outcomes may be more broadly defined than others. The anticipated desired outcomes should be defined because they can vary considerably even with one single intervention; for instance, the outcome following coronary artery bypass surgery may be measured in terms of in-hospital mortality rates, 30-day mortality rates or relief of angina at 1, 5 or 10 years. The desired outcomes should be defined by the existing medical literature and an in-depth knowledge of the impact of the intervention.

However, the full range of outcomes that will arise as a consequence of an intervention is not always known. Outcomes can be grouped into the following categories: unexpected, expected and unpredictable. The latter category would include events that occur because of care or despite care and may be positive or negative. There may also be varying degrees of certainty in terms of anticipating outcomes (e.g. a large amount of potassium chloride given intravenously will cause cardiac arrest) and in other instances it may not be known what the outcomes of care will be, e.g. with treatment such as new chemotherapy, it may be difficult to anticipate the outcome benefit with any great certainty.

Outcome instrument, measure or indicator?

Confusion can and does develop when the terms 'indicator', 'instrument' and 'measure' are used to mean different things, a phenomenon which does prevail throughout the literature (Fries 1983, Shaw 1986, Marek 1989). While a great deal of the literature refers to 'outcome measures', 'outcome indicators' or 'outcome instruments', the term 'outcome' has also been used in isolation to imply:

- data-collecting tool (e.g. questionnaire, checklist);
- the dimension of health status under investigation (e.g. functional status, well-being);
- the validity of the dimension of health status under investigation.

The terms 'outcome instrument', 'measure' and 'indicator' have all been used synonymously and differently within the literature. Brettle (1995), for instance, claims that the term 'outcome instrument' can be referred to as a measure or an indicator. This implies that all three terms are similar in nature and perform similar functions. This viewpoint is justified on the basis that the term 'outcome indicator' is used to imply the dimension of health status (e.g. functional status), while 'instrument' is used to denote the tool used to collect information on the dimension of health under investigation, e.g. questionnaires and satisfaction surveys. Other authors use the term 'outcome measure' as an umbrella term to denote the data collection tool and also to refer to the dimension of health status under investigation (Higgins et al 1992).

Others have described the concepts differently. Williams (1991) considers an indicator to be ' ... a numerical representation of the evaluation of the structure, process or outcomes of care'. The Joint Commission on Accreditation of Health Care Organisations (1989), as cited by Williams (1991), describes an indicator as being either a sentinel event indicator or rate-based indicator. A sentinel event indicator identifies a grave untoward process or outcome of care. Usually, and ideally, the incidence of this type of indicator will remain low (e.g. pressure sores). A rate-based indicator identifies patient care outcomes or processes of care that may require further assessment based on significant trending or variances from thresholds over time (i.e. percentage of patients prepared for discharge). Hutchinson et al (1996) use the term 'outcome indicator' as a measure of health that can be used quantitatively to describe the health of a group of people in a particular setting (such as general practice or an outpatient clinic). This is in contrast to the Joint Commission on Accreditation of Health Care Organisations (1989) whose recommendations clearly stipulate that it does not consider an indicator to be a measure of health.

HEALTH OUTCOME ASSESSMENT IN PRACTICE

The main reasons for establishing an outcome initiative have been summarised in a consensus statement (Davis et al 1994) and include the following three areas:

1. to describe in quantitative terms the impact of care on patients' lives;
2. to establish a reliable basis for clinical decision making by clinicians and patients; and
3. to evaluate the effectiveness of care and identify opportunities for improvement.

There may be many factors influencing a person's health, yet only some are related to the care received by that individual. If the outcome measures are used to judge performance, then there must be some relationship between the activities of the health-care provision and the resultant patient or population outcome (Faust et al 1997). One of the key problems is the fact that there are many influences on health and that it may not be possible to identify realistic improvements in health that can be attributed specifically to a particular intervention. The uncertainty of the links between the process and outcome of health care is a recurrent problem (Mullins et al 1996) although there is agreement that an outcome measure should reflect the objectives of care.

In the Outcome Measures in Ambulatory Care Study (McColl et al 1995), criteria were identified that related to the practical issues of outcome assessment acknowledging that this aspect was as important as the scientific rigour in their development. The project team concluded that for outcome assessment to be a routine part of clinical practice, the method had to satisfy some basic criteria:

• inexpensive and simple methods of data collection;
• unobtrusive to patient care;
• able to generate clear feedback in a meaningful time frame;
• relevant and appropriate scientific basis.

APPROACHES TO HEALTH OUTCOME ASSESSMENT

The focus extends from a macro perspective, i.e. a set of all-embracing influences on health (e.g. social, environmental, political and employment factors), through to a micro perspective, i.e. a set of outcomes emanating from specific influences from a clearly identified group of services (e.g. nursing interventions). The three levels of outcome considered by Hegyvary (1992) are as follows.

1. *Macro level* – Outcomes are focused on the health of populations and are related not only to the health-care system but also to environmental influences such as unemployment and poverty (e.g. the health of the over-65s may be an example of a macro-level outcome indicator).

2. *Meso level* – defined in terms of the impact of interventions directed to a specific client group, e.g. the functional abilities of clients who have undergone coronary artery bypass surgery, are influenced by clinical and organisational variables.

3. *Micro level* – refers to individual responses to particular interventions, such as drug therapies.

Macro level

The government has set out targets for health improvement that will be used in outcome assessment of multiagency, intersectoral activities to improve health (DoH 1998, DoH in Scotland 1999). It recognises that many factors can influence health and has an overarching focus on tackling health inequalities. Life circumstances, as reflected by a worthwhile job, decent housing, good education and a clean and pleasant environment, make for physical and mental well-being. Changes in these factors should be reflected in the type of outcome assessment measures used to monitor change. This has not been made explicit in the documentation and targets for outcome assessment focus on decreased mortality in specific disease areas and improvements in behavioural lifestyle factors. Four priority areas have been identified as follows:

1. heart disease and stroke;
2. accidents;
3. cancer;
4. mental health.

These have been selected because they are significant causes of premature death and poor health and much can be done to prevent them or to treat them more effectively. There are marked inequalities across socioeconomic groups in society and effective outcome measures should reflect changes in inequalities in life circumstances. The targets for outcome assessment for these priority areas are presented in Box 12.1.

Meso and micro levels

Structured health measures have been developed to offer an insight into subjective aspects of health that are not easily ascertained from population statistics, such as hospital utilisation and mortality figures. They are useful in assessing both health need and outcome as a result of health-care intervention. They rely on the judgement of individuals and therefore are subjective. Although reports on health are not inherently quantitative, the results and scores obtained from responses are translated into quantitative estimates. Typically these instruments consist of a set of closed questions which have a limited number of responses and the respondents have to take those closest to their own view. Some form of rating method is utilised to translate the statement into a numerical estimate of the different dimensions of health being assessed so that the responses can be analysed statistically.

Box 12.1 Outcome targets for the period 1995–2010

Coronary heart disease
- Reduce premature mortality by 50%

Cancer
- Reduce premature mortality by 20%

Smoking
- Reduce smoking among 12–15-year-olds from 14% to 11%
- Reduce the proportion of women smoking during pregnancy from 29% to 20%

Alcohol misuse
- Reduce the incidence of men and women exceeding weekly limits from 33% to 29% and 13% to 11% respectively

Teenage pregnancy
- Reduce rate among 13–15-year-olds by 20%

Dental health
- 60% of 5-year-old children with no experience of dental disease

Accidents
- Reduce by 20% the rate of accidents as defined by an accident that results in a hospital visit or consultation with a family doctor

Mental health
- Reduce the death rate from suicide and undetermined injury by 17%

Health inequalities
- National targets remain to be defined. Commitment to monitor initiatives aimed at tackling health problems in neighbourhoods or groups that suffer from poorer health, in addition to the whole population

---

In the interpretation of responses generated from health assessment questionnaires, their inherent subjectiveness should be remembered, not least because individuals with and without disease have different health experiences. The importance of obtaining a quantitative estimate of level of health has been described as most useful when used as a comparative entity rather than an absolute state in itself (Smith 1981). In terms of health status measurement in practice, comparisons of health states between groups of individuals and of the same individuals before and after interventions are the most common usage of assessment.

Reliability and validity

Reliability of the measure or questionnaire being used is concerned with its ability to obtain the same results when used repeatedly in a similar situation or setting. Test–retest reliability is used to establish the extent to which a measure, when administered to an individual twice under identical conditions, produces agreement between the two sets of responses. However, because health or the symptoms related to a particular condition may change over time, it is not a straightforward process to determine whether differences recorded using a particular measure are a weakness in the measure itself or whether changes that have occurred are being picked up. A knowledge of expected variance in health and in particular conditions is necessary to interpret changes observed and to make an informed judgement on the sources of any changes observed.

Validity is a measure of the tool's ability to accurately assess the area under enquiry (Oppenheim 1992). Health itself is a complex, abstract and variable entity which depends on the perspective from which it is viewed and this causes difficulty in the establishment of validity. The validity of an instrument refers to the extent to which the indicator measures the desired underlying concept. The questions should be unambiguous, easily understood and reflect issues that are appropriate. Items should reflect a comprehensive overview of the attribute being measured. *Construct validity* examines the relationship between underlying theoretical issues and the measure. It relies on a proper theoretical basis for the particular measurement. This can be problematic when the theoretical basis is health, which relies on many different theoretical perspectives. *Criterion validity* refers to the extent to which the measure correlates with a preexisting one, preferably a 'gold standard'. However, there may not be such a measure available and, in some instances, more than one health status measurement may be utilised.

Responsiveness

Responsiveness or sensitivity to change refers to the ability of an outcome measure to detect change in health status between the same health states in different individuals and in the same individuals over time. In order to establish the responsiveness of a measure to change, a comparison should be made with another ideally 'gold standard' measure of the same attribute under assessment. The problem inherent in this process is often the lack of an appropriate 'gold standard'. The changes recorded by an outcome measure should reflect genuine changes in the dimension of health status under observation.

GENERIC AND DISEASE-SPECIFIC HEALTH MEASUREMENT INSTRUMENTS

There are two broad classifications of tools or measures designed to assess health status: the generic measure and the disease-specific measure (Donovan et al 1993, Guyatt et al 1993).

Generic instruments

Generic instruments assess a spectrum of quality of life components or domains and are applicable to a variety of populations. They also allow for comparisons of health status across different disease states and patient groups (Oldridge 1997). A generic tool would be the preferred measure when comparing health levels in a general population or in a variety of disease states. The generic health-care measures can be criticised on the basis that they need to be broadly comprehensive in order to cover all conditions and diseases but in so doing, they may fail to measure the specific and important impairments associated with any one condition. In addition, there is growing evidence that some generic measures may not be responsive to small but important changes when used to assess effective interventions (Anderson et al 1993).

The Short-Form 36 Health Questionnaire

The Short-Form 36 (SF-36) (Ware et al 1993) is a general health questionnaire that was developed in the United States from a larger inventory of questions designed to measure health status. It has now been adapted for use in the UK and other European countries and has been used extensively in healthy population groups and with patients with specific conditions.

Multiple categories of operational health definitions were selected to measure both physical and mental health in terms of behavioural functioning; perceived well-being; social and role disability; personal perceptions of health in general. The resultant SF-36 was a 36-item scale generating scores for eight health dimensions, namely physical functioning, role limitation due to physical health problems, bodily pain, general health, vitality (energy/fatigue), social functioning, role limitations due to emotional problems and mental health (psychological distress and psychological well-being). The scores for each domain are based on the same scale of 0–100 where 0 is the worst possible health status and 100 the optimum. Previous work utilising this health status measure has found that it may be unable to detect clinically important changes for individuals whose health is either very poor or very good.

The Nottingham Health Profile

The Nottingham Health Profile (Hunt & McEwen 1980, 1985) is a multi-dimensional measure of health which was developed through the utilisation of patients' perception and language rather than medical judgements and categories. It is similar to the Sickness Impact Profile (Bergner et al 1981) with its focus on the impact of disease on that individual, although the Sickness Impact Profile focuses on the behavioural consequences of disease. The Nottingham Health Profile (NHP) asks about feelings and emotional state directly.

Reports on a variety of aspects of acute and chronic ailments were obtained from patients. A system of weighting responses was developed and groups of patients and non-patients were asked to compare statements and make judgements on severity. The NHP consists of two parts which can be used independently. Part one consists of 38 statements grouped into six sections: mobility, pain, sleep, social isolation, emotional reaction and energy. Part two of the questionnaire asks respondents to indicate whether or not their state of health affects activity in seven areas of daily life. These include employment, looking after the home, social life, home life, sex life, interests and hobbies, and holidays. Responses are coded as a simple 'yes' or 'no' and no weighting is provided for the different items.

The NHP is suitable for individuals or groups of people over the age of 16 and has been used in populations of elderly, fit and ill people as well as general population samples. However, it is not truly a measure of health but more a measure of distress as a result of ill health. Its content seems more suited to people suffering from chronic illnesses rather than to general populations or those suffering from minor health problems.

The Sickness Impact Profile

The Sickness Impact Profile (SIP) (Bergner et al 1981) is a measure of sickness-related behavioural dysfunction as judged by the individual's perception of the impact of the illness on usual daily activities. It was developed in the United States and was designed to be applicable across types and severities of illness and within demographic and cultural subgroups.

The objective of the authors was to create a general-purpose measure of the impact of disease. The concept of sickness, which denotes the individual's experience of illness through its effect on everyday life and feelings, is contrasted with the medical model of disease, which denotes a professional-based definition of clinical observations. Aspects of behaviour included in the profile were selected because they represented what were considered to be universal patterns of limitations that may be affected by any illness regardless of the specific condition.

An initial large pool of statements were finally reduced to 136 statements in 12 categories, including sleep and rest, eating, work, home management, recreation and pastimes, ambulation, mobility, body care and movement, social interaction and communication. A panel of judges, including professional and lay perspectives, rated each of the items from minimally dysfunctional to maximum dysfunction to represent the relative severity of limitation on behaviour implied by each statement.

The SIP has been used in a wide variety of populations and individual groups but has been particularly useful in studies of patients suffering from chronic illness. It is well documented and has been widely used in the US but less so in the UK. However, its length may make it impractical for use in many situations, particularly at population level. In addition, because of its general purpose and design to be reliable and valid across a wide variety of groups, it may be less responsive to significant clinical changes over time in the same individuals.

Disease-specific measures

Disease-specific measures are useful in the context of one disease entity where health status may be affected by a range of symptoms related to a particular condition or disease. Specific instruments focus on problems associated with single disease states, patient groups or areas of function (Guyatt et al 1993). Specific measures concentrate on particular conditions or populations. A growing number of researchers find it necessary to use, in addition to generic health status measures, disease-specific measurements in order to capture the specific quality of life issues associated with the condition of interest (Marks et al 1992, Juniper et al 1993). The strength of disease-specific instruments lies in their ability to focus on the areas of function that have been considered most important to patients in relation to the symptoms and effects of the condition (McDowell & Newell 1987). Their limitation is that the degree of impairment cannot be compared across different conditions. It is generally appreciated that individuals with and without disease have different health experiences.

The Hospital Anxiety and Depression Scale

The Hospital Anxiety and Depression Scale (Zigmond & Snaith 1983) has been designed to detect the presence and severity of relatively mild degrees of mood disorder, likely to be found in non-psychiatric hospital outpatients. It was intended both as a screening tool and as a method of charting progress over time. The scale consists of 14 items, seven of which relate to depression and seven to anxiety. There is a mixture of questions formed in the positive and negative wording. Responses relate to feelings during the last week and respondents are encouraged to give their immediate reaction rather than a carefully considered answer. The questions for the depression subscale concentrate on loss of pleasure as this is a key indicator used in monitoring the effectiveness of antidepressant therapy. Items for the anxiety subscale are a summary of the author's own research into the psychological manifestations of anxiety neurosis.

The scale had been used in a wide variety of patients suffering from chronic conditions such as rheumatoid arthritis, respiratory problems, inflammatory bowel disease, cancer and early dementia. It is recommended for use in adults between the ages of 16 and 65 with further research recommended for use in elderly patients. It is short and self-administered and in the absence of reference to symptoms which might be attributable to physical illness, it makes a tool well suited for use in primary health care. Although its focus is narrow, it is important because anxiety and depression are by far the most common problems seen in primary health care and as such, it is well worth consideration.

The Arthritis Impact Measurement Scale

The Arthritis Impact Measurement Scale (AIMS) (Meenan et al 1980) has been designed to measure the health status component of patient outcome in rheumatic diseases and has been used to evaluate various treatments and programmes, both in clinical research and in service evaluation. The authors recognise that the WHO definition of health should constitute the criteria for outcome evaluation and provide the theoretical basis through which the instrument should be built. In addition, they drew on several other established scales of health and well-being and physical and mental health to provide the core elements for the AIMS and included new measurements related to pain and dexterity.

The core elements for each section include mobility, dexterity, pain, activities of daily living, social activity, household activity, depression and anxiety. Scores have been shown to correlate well with age and patients' perception of their general health and it is likely to be of particular value in studies of rheumatic diseases in general practice or as a routine adjunct to clinical practice, both in needs assessment and in outcomes of care intervention.

The McGill Pain Questionnaire

The McGill Pain Questionnaire (Melzack 1975, 1983) was designed to provide quantifiable measures of clinical pain and was originally intended to provide a means of detecting differences among different methods of relieving pain and, to a lesser extent, has been used in diagnostic differentiation. The author pointed out that his conception of pain was more than a single sensation that varies only in intensity and included a variety of qualities that could be categorised under the heading of pain. Three major classes of terminology were used in their classification: words that describe sensory qualities, words that describe affective qualities and evaluative words. Groups of doctors' patients and students were asked to assign intensity values to each word using a numerical scale. After eliminating areas of disagreement and consolidating areas of consensus, the instrument was developed and piloted and although there was agreement that further research was required, it has not been conducted and the instrument is used on the basis of the early developmental work.

There are at least five versions of this questionnaire, including a longer and short version. The standard version has been used in a wide variety of patient groups, including those suffering from low back pain, arthritis, headache, cancer and postoperative pain. Although there are a number of alternative pain measures available, the McGill Pain Questionnaire is the most widely used. It is preferable to simpler measures of pain intensity because it recognises the complexity of the experience and is based on a clear theoretical formulation of this.

SOCIAL ASPECTS OF HEALTH

The social model of health is discussed in detail in Chapter 3. Social exclusion has been recognised at health policy level as a contributing factor to ill health and a target for health improvement initiatives (DoH 1998). In order to assess progress in this area, tools to assess outcome will be useful. Several instruments have been developed and are summarised by Wilkin et al (1992). The Social Activities Questionnaire is worthy of inclusion in this chapter because of its brevity and ease of use in practice although it is limited by its major focus on quantitative aspects of social contacts with less assessment of the nature and intrinsic personal value of relationships.

Social Activities Questionnaire

The Social Activities Questionnaire was developed as a measure of social well-being for use in the Rand Health Insurance Experiment (Lohr et al 1986a, 1986b). It was based on the concept that social well-being had two distinct dimensions related to quality and quantity. Quantity was concerned with the number of contacts and the amount of activity whereas quality was concerned with personal evaluations of the meaning and satisfaction of interpersonal relationships. The selection of questions was based on the adaptation of a number of existing instruments (Donald & Ware 1982), to meet a range of specified criteria including conceptual relevance, variability in score distribution, repeatability and sensitivity to the effects of medical care (Myers et al 1975, Donald et al 1978). Item scaling was accomplished by examining the relationships between responses to each item and the three variables of emotional ties, psychological well-being and current health.

There are 11 items in the scale covering social contacts, group participation, social activities and subjective evaluation of the quality of relationships. Response categories can be converted into scale scores for each item and an overall summary index of social support calculated. The higher the score, the greater the level of social support and typically scores range from 8 to 40. The score is used as a relative measure of social support rather than an absolute measure in itself.

CONCLUSION

In summary, this chapter has explored the use of the terminology associated with 'outcomes'. In particular, the review has highlighted both the diversity of interpretations and applications of the terminology associated with outcomes. In describing the manner in which the terminology has been applied, the review has illustrated the sometimes inconsistent approach to the use of terms such as 'patient or nursing outcome' or 'instrument', 'indicator' or 'measure'. Although consensus regarding these definitions has not yet been reached, exploring the complexities of terms and concepts has highlighted the many variables that impinge on the outcome of care for an individual and for the health of a population.

In the primary care-led NHS, general practitioner and health authority commissioners have responsibility for evaluating the effectiveness of health care. Comparisons of health outcome between different patterns of primary health care have been limited due to the lack of an outcome measure sensitive to change and with the ability to adjust for differences in case mix. Changes in health functioning in the hypothesised directions with age, employment grade, social and economic status and disease status are important considerations for judging the sensitivity of an outcome instrument. It will be important for users who wish to apply such outcome instruments over time in the same individuals to examine and establish the responsiveness. This can be done by testing a measure on patients receiving treatment where treatment effects are well established and quantifiable and assessing the capability of the measure in detecting these treatment effects.

Measures of health outcome have been less extensively used in primary health care than in other specialities. Multidimensional measures for large population groups are likely to be the most relevant for use in general practice but it should be recognised that they are unlikely to include sufficient detail to evaluate care of certain major chronic illnesses, for example arthritis, bronchitis, diabetes and coronary heart disease. Thus, disease-specific measures have their place in areas where there is lack of clarity of responsiveness and sensitivity to change in specific patient groups. In the interpretation of results from the use of such instrumentation, it will also be necessary to assess inputs other than direct patient care to include services such as social support, the environment, economic circumstances and broader life situation.

There is increasing awareness of the need within a complex health-care system to both maximise effectiveness and establish efficacy and efficiency. Monitoring needs for and outcomes of care is essential to this process and this is reflected in the increasing trend for the use of audits as a means of monitoring care. The effectiveness of such audits will be dependent on the tools used. Continued development and evaluation will be necessary, not least to take into account patients' needs to ensure they are met and that desirable outcomes are achieved.

REFERENCES

Anderson R T, Aaronson N K, Wilkin D 1993 Critical review of the international assessments of health-related quality of life. Quality of Life Research 2: 369–395

Barriball K L, MacKenzie A 1993 Measuring the impact of nursing interventions in the community: a selective review of the literature. Journal of Advanced Nursing 18: 401–407

Bergner M, Bobbitt R A, Carter W B, Gilson B S 1981 The Sickness Impact Profile: development and final version of a health status measure. Medical Care 19: 787–805

Bloch D 1975 Evaluation of nursing care in terms of process and outcome: issues in research and quality assurance. Nursing Research 24(4): 256–263

Bond S 1992 Outcomes of nursing: proceedings of an invitational developmental workshop. University of Newcastle, Newcastle upon Tyne

Bond S, Thomas L H 1992 Measuring patients' satisfaction with nursing care. Journal of Advanced Nursing 17: 52–63

Brettle A 1995 Outcome instruments for nurses: how to find out more about them. Nurse Researcher 2(4): 14–29

Brook R H, Williams K N, Avery A D 1976 Quality assurance today and tomorrow: forecast for the future. Annals of Internal Medicine 85: 809–817

Burback F R, Quarry A 1991 Quality and outcome in a community mental health team. International Journal of Health Care and Quality Assurance 4(2): 18–26

Clark J 1983 Evaluating health visiting practice. Health Visitor 56(6): 205–208

Davis A R, Doyle M A, Lansky D, Rutt W, Orsolitis S, Doyle J B 1994 Outcomes assessment in clinical settings: a consensus statement on principles and best practices in project management. Joint Commission Journal on Quality Improvement 20(1): 6–16

Del Bueno D 1993 Outcome evaluation: frustration or fertile field? Journal of Nursing Administration 23(7/8): 12–19

DoH 1998 Our healthier nation: a contract for health. Stationery Office, London

DoH in Scotland 1999 Towards a healthier Scotland. Stationery Office, Edinburgh

Doll R, Peto R, Wheatley K, Gray R, Sutherland L 1994 Mortality in relation to smoking: 40 years' observation on male British doctors. British Medical Journal 309: 901–911

Donabedian A 1966 Evaluating the quality of care. Millbank Memorial Fund Quarterly 44(2): 166–206

Donabedian A 1969 Some issues in evaluating the quality of nursing care. American Journal of Public Health 59(10): 1833–1836

Donabedian A 1980 The definition of quality and approaches to its management. Explorations in quality assessment and monitoring. Health Administration Press, Ann Arbor, MI

Donabedian A 1989 Institutional and professional responsibilities in quality assurance. Quality Assurance in Health Care 1(1): 3–11

Donald C A, Ware J E 1982 The quantification of social contacts and resources. Rand Corporation, Santa Monica, CA

Donald C A, Ware J E, Brook R H, Davies-Avery A 1978 Conceptualization and measurement of health for adults in the Health Insurance Study. R-1987/4 HEW. Rand Corporation, Santa Monica, CA

Donovan J L, Frankel S J, Eyles J D 1993 Assessing the need for health status measures. Journal of Epidemiology and Community Health 47: 158–162

Faust H B, Mirowski G W, Chuang T Y et al 1997 Outcomes research: an overview. Journal of the American Academy of Dermatology 36(6,1): 999–1006

Fries J M 1983 Toward an understanding of patient outcome measurement. Arthritis and Rheumatism 26(6): 697–704

Guyatt G H, Feeney D H, Patrick D L 1993 Measuring health related quality of life: basic sciences review. Annals of Internal Medicine 118: 622–629

Hegyvary S T 1992 Outcomes research: integrating nursing practice into the world view. In: Patient outcomes research: examining the effectiveness of nursing practice. Proceedings of a conference sponsored by the National Center for Nursing Research. US Department of Health and Human Services, Washington DC

Higgins M, McCaughan D, Griffiths M, Carr-Hill R 1992 Assessing the outcomes of nursing care. Journal of Advanced Nursing 17(5): 561–568

Hunt S, McEwen J 1980 The development of a subjective health indicator. Social Health and Illness 2(3): 231–246

Hunt S, McEwen J 1985 Measuring health status: a new tool for clinicians and epidemiologists. Journal of the Royal College of General Practitioners 35: 185–188

Hutchinson A, McColl E, Christie M, Riccalton C (eds) 1996 Health outcome measures in primary and out-patient care. Harwood Academic Publishers, Amsterdam

Jennings B M 1991 Patient outcomes research: seizing the opportunity. Advances in Nurse Science 14(2): 59–72

Joint Commission on Accreditation of Health Care Organisations 1989 Characteristics of clinical indicators. Quality Review Bulletin 15(11): 330–339

Juniper E F, Guyatt G H, Ferrie P J, Griffith L E 1993 Measuring quality of life in asthma. American Review of Respiratory Disease 147: 832–838

Lohr K N 1988 Outcome measurement: concepts and questions. Inquiry 25(1): 37–50

Lohr K N, Brook R H, Kamberg C J et al 1986a Use of medical care in the Rand Health Insurance Experiment. Diagnosis- and service-specific analyses in a randomized controlled trial. Medical Care 24: S1–S7

Lohr K N, Kamberg C J, Keeler E B, Goldberg G A, Calabro T A, Brook R H 1986b Chronic disease in a general adult population. Findings from the Rand Health Insurance Experiment. Western Journal of Medicine 145: 537–545

Long A F, Dixon P, Hall R, Carr-Hill R A, Sheldon T A 1993 The outcomes agenda: contribution of the UK clearing house on health outcomes. Quality in Health Care 2: 49–52

Marek K D 1989 Outcome measurement in nursing. Journal of Nursing and Quality Assurance 4(1): 1–9

Marks G B, Dunn S M, Woolcock A J 1992 A scale for the measurement of quality of life in adults with asthma. Journal of Clinical Epidemiology 45: 461–472

McColl E, Steen I N, Meadows K A et al 1995 Developing outcome measures for ambulatory care: an application to asthma and diabetes. Social Science and Medicine 41(10): 1339–1348

McDowell I, Newell C 1987 Measuring health: a guide to rating scales and questionnaires. Oxford University Press, New York

Meenan R F, Gertman P M, Manson J H 1980 Measuring health status in arthritis: the Arthritis Impact Measurement Scales. Arthritis and Rheumatism 23: 146–152

Melzack R 1975 The McGill Pain Questionnaire: major properties and scoring methods. Pain 11: 93–100

Melzack R (ed) 1983 Pain measurement and assessment. Raven Press, New York

Myers J K, Lindenthal J J, Pepper M P 1975 Life events, social integration and psychiatric symptomatology. Journal of Health and Social Behaviour 16: 421–427

Mullins C D, Baldwin R, Perfetto E M 1996 What are outcomes? Journal of the American Pharmaceutical Association 36(1): 39–49

Nightingale F 1859 Notes on nursing: what it is and what it is not. Harrison, London

Norman I, Redfern S 1993 The quality of nursing. Nursing Times 89(27): 40–43

Oldridge N B 1997 Outcome assessment in cardiac rehabilitation. Health-related quality of life and economic evaluation. Journal of Cardiopulmonary Rehabilitation 17: 179–194

Oppenheim A 1992 Questionnaire design – interviewing and attitude measurement, 2nd edn. Pinter, London

Shanks J, Frater A 1993 Health status, outcome, and attributability: is a red rose red in the dark? Quality in Health Care 2: 259–262

Shaw C D 1986 Introducing quality assurance. King's Fund Project Paper 64. King's Fund, London

Smith J A 1981 The idea of health: a philosophical inquiry. Advances in Nursing Science 3 (3): 43–50

Van Maanen H M 1981 Improvement of quality of nursing care: a goal to challenge in the eighties. Journal of Advanced Nursing 6: 3–6

Ware J, Snow K K, Kosinski M, Gandek B 1993 SF36 Health Survey: manual and interpretation guide. The Health Institute, New England Medical Centre, Boston, MA

Waters K 1986 Cause and effect. Nursing Times 82(5): 28–30

Wilkin D, Hallam L, Doggett M-A 1992 Measures of need and outcome for primary health care. Oxford University Press, Oxford

Williams A D 1991 Development and application of clinical indicators for nursing. Journal of Nursing Care Quality 6(1): 1–5

Zigmond A S, Snaith R P 1983 The Hospital Anxiety and Depression Scale. Acta Psychiatra Scandinavica 67: 361–370

13

Health-care policy making

Stephen Peckham

INTRODUCTION

The last 15 years have seen some fundamental changes in UK health-care policy which have had important implications for the nursing contribution to public health. Many of these developments have already been discussed in previous chapters on nursing, commissioning and primary care. This chapter discusses the broad sweep of these health-care policy changes as they relate to nursing and public health. The election of a Labour government in 1997 had important consequences for the development of health-care policy and particular attention is paid to recent developments in primary care and public health policy. While primary care policy can be seen as building on policy developments from 1991 onwards, public health policy appears to have shifted significantly in its focus from the previous government's approach in the 1980s and early 1990s.

While the principal aim of this chapter is to provide a context for public health nursing as we enter the new millennium, it will also examine ways in which nurses can influence debate about public health and engage in the policy-making process. The chapter will therefore be more than a review of health-care policy. It begins by outlining the health-care policy-making process in the UK and examines some of the ways in which nurses can become involved in health-care policy making. Thus the chapter picks up on themes in earlier chapters about what a public health role for nurses really means within the context of the UK health-care system. That nurses, both as individual practitioners and as a profession, should influence policy and practice has to be a key strategic goal for, as Spurgeon (1997) has argued, a more autonomous and empowered profession, and professional, is likely to lead to more effective working and levels of satisfaction.

HEALTH POLICY-MAKING PROCESS
Introduction

The study of policy making is in itself a whole academic discipline which has developed particularly in the postwar period. It is not therefore my intention to explore the policy-making process in great detail as this has been done elsewhere (Harrison et al 1990, Ham 1992). My aim here is to introduce the main principles of policy making in the UK NHS and explore who is involved. As outlined above, there are some key themes which run within the NHS since its establishment in 1948 and distinct trends can be identified within these themes which are relevant to both our understanding of the NHS and to examining how it is possible to influence health policy.

These interactions will be explored further below but first it is important to define what policy is.

What is policy?

Policy has variously been described as a course of action or inaction, a web of decisions, a set of interrelated decisions which seek to allocate resources or select goals and the means of achieving them (Ham & Hill 1984). Thus, a definition of policy is beset with difficulties. So how would we recognise health policy? Clearly, formal declarations of policy are contained in official government documents such as the White Paper *The new NHS* or pronouncements in Parliament. However, policies such as *The new NHS* change through implementation. Thus policy intent is insufficient to identify what occurs, i.e. what changes are brought about. So, in examining what policy is, we must also be concerned with the process of policy making and policy implementation.

The need to address implementation is particularly relevant to health policy due to the extent and rapidity of organisational changes in the 1990s; in particular, the fragmentation of the NHS which has brought with it both greater decentralisation and centralisation (Klein 1995).

Usefully, Frenk (1994) has described four levels of the policy process.

- The *systematic level* is that which shapes the health system overall – policy on the way the NHS or public health is structured and organised.
- The *programmatic level* is concerned with deciding health priorities and resource allocation at the macro level such as HA decisions on funding for children's services or mental health.

- The *organisational level* is concerned with the way health services operate such as the organisation and management of PCGs and their relations with other providers.
- The *instrumental level* is where management policy is made and relates much more to implementation.

While there is some separation between these different levels of policy process, in reality aspects of each of these levels can be seen operating both nationally and locally. Certainly, decisions about the overall shape of the NHS are taken at national level but some organisational policy is also made nationally. In order to explore this more, it is necessary to look at how policy is made.

How is health policy made?

There is no simple answer to this question and there has been much written on this subject. Essentially, policy is seen as a rational response to a given problem. However, in practice the process is more complex and messy, leading to concepts of incrementalism, where policy develops on a 'muddling through' basis, and mixed scanning, where policy is developed through an exploration of potential options. However, these theories of policy making do not provide an adequate account of what happens where it is often difficult to see why particular issues find their way onto policy agendas.

As suggested above, current health policy is based on previous experience – the continuity of developing policy over a long period of time such as a primary care-led NHS and increasing managerialism. This is the idea of social learning and is associated with the concept of incremental change, making small changes in an incremental way rather than large policy shifts. However, on its own, social learning is insufficient to explain policy changes. For example, when examining the introduction of the internal market in the NHS in 1991 it is difficult to see this as an incremental change. Thus we also need to look to ideological changes such as an attachment to market-based approaches or, more recently, the reemphasis on inequalities within public health policy, central to the current government's approach.

Finally, policy is about what is possible and even ideological shifts can be muted by the art of the possible. For example, in the debates over reform in the late 1980s, privatisation of the health service was quickly ruled out as not being politically possible. Policy therefore develops from the interplay of social learning and ideology with a touch of realism – rather like mixing a soup. This suggests that the policy process involves a wide range of actors who become involved at one or more of the four levels described above.

However, there has been a distinct change in the policy process over the last 50 years (Harrison & Wood 1999). In the 1960s and 1970s the approach to policy development was much more detailed with the establishment of royal commissions or detailed planning bodies, such as for the Hospital Plan (MoH 1962) and the 1974 reorganisation (DHSS 1971). By the 1980s the policy development was much less detailed (see the Griffiths reports on management and community care). Over the last 10 years much policy has only provided a sketchy outline with detailed policy developed as you go along (e.g. fundholding and PCG guidance). There may be a number of reasons for this, including increasing complexity of the organisation of health care, difficulties in ensuring policy compliance and the need to develop quick responses (Harrison & Wood 1999). One consequence is that there may be more opportunities to influence the final shape of local provision where policy requires further development.

Who makes policy?

Such a question may appear very simple for surely it is the government who makes policy. However, you may have realised from the discussion above and elsewhere in this book that it is not only government who makes policy. In relation to health care, some key policies are developed by the professional bodies, such as the UKCC which sets standards for nurse training and practice which are nationally applicable and thus are significant policies. Health and local authorities also make policies. For example, in recent years rationing policies have been a key focus of debate within HAs. We also need to examine the role of the civil service – the bureaucrats in the Department of Health and the NHS Executive – pressure groups, including professional associations such as the RCN and CPHVA, the media, Parliament, political parties and other central government departments such as the Treasury.

Thus, we have a long list of potential contributors to the policy process. This is the policy community – the range of actors who are involved in shaping policy. Not all actors have equal say in the policy process. You might expect that the government would have the most say but this is too simplistic. In health policy, particularly in relation to health-care services, professional organisations such as the BMA and royal colleges have enormous power. These provider interest groups have been involved in policy development and implementation since the inception of the NHS (Williamson 1992).

INFLUENCING PUBLIC HEALTH POLICY

As suggested above, the new framework for health-care commissioning and public health provides some new opportunities for nurses to influence the development and practice of public health. Central to this is the commitment to the development of public health strategy at a local (health authority) level and the role of nursing in primary care commissioning outlined in the White and Green Papers. These opportunities are firmly within a local policy-making context. However, public health requires a national context as well. This is explicitly recognised within *Our healthier nation* which sets out the key roles for national government. Hennessy (1997) suggests that:

Many nurses are in positions to participate in the policy process, either by influencing policies as they are made or by getting involved with the implementation. Whatever the level of their involvement, nurses have to understand the policy processes so that correct actions can be taken at the appropriate time. (p. 37)

Peter Spurgeon (1997) has argued that currently nurses are more operationally focused and that few are active in the policy arena. This is evidenced by the profession's and NHS's slow response to defining the nursing role in commissioning during the 1990s. While in relation to the development of *The new NHS* the profession has clearly won a major policy goal in the inclusion of primary care nurses on PCG boards, it is not clear what role they should play or what their constituency should be. At the same time, however, such developments open up new possibilities for influencing local commissioning policy.

   Despite this, there are many questions about the interrelationship of these organisational policies and the public health agenda (Peckham et al 1998). How can nurses influence this national agenda and in what ways will it be possible to affect local health policy and the implementation of public health policy? In order to help nurses make sense of the local and national opportunities, the next two sections of this chapter will outline the local and national contexts of policy making and provide some suggestions on how you can become engaged in public health policy development and implementation. Each section provides an outline of how and where policy making occurs and how nurses could become engaged with these processes. The sections also provide pointers to key organisations and associations through which nurses may influence the public health debate as well as public health policy and action.

National frameworks

As has been discussed above, key policy is made at a national level by the government. This is a consequence of both the nature of the NHS but also the wider policy processes that operate in the UK. However, policy is not made in a vacuum and it evolves from a complex set of circumstances and inputs from those within the government and civil service but also from outside agencies. There are a number of ways in which nurses can become involved in this process.

The first is to try and influence the opinions and decisions made by the government through political pressure via elections and political parties. The limitations of general elections are obvious but there are some distinct differences between political parties on how to tackle public health issues. Second, party political membership and activity can provide a conduit for influencing party policy. Alternatively you can use your MP to raise questions in Parliament and request information from relevant departments. It should be recognised, though, that these methods of influencing policy at a national level have only limited success although they can help put specific topics on to the national political agenda.

Another approach is through national professional organisations who attempt to influence government policy. Provider interests have always been more prominent in influencing health policy than other interests. Thus, the roles of the RCN, Royal College of Midwives and the Community Practitioners and Health Visiting Association (CPHVA) are very important. Both the RCN and CPHVA have strong interests in public health issues and actively seek to influence the national policy agenda by direct engagement with leading policy makers in the government, Department of Health, NHS Executive and other relevant government departments. They operate individually but also in alliances with other professional bodies and public health interest groups. It is perhaps more useful, therefore, for nurses to become actively involved in their professional organisations if they wish to influence national policy debates. These associations form policy networks. The key groups in national policy networks are shown in Figure 13.1 and a list of some of the main national public health organisations and professional organisations is given in the Useful Addresses Section at the end of the book.

Before examining local policy stakeholders, it is necessary to consider briefly the impact of devolution. The development of the Scottish Parliament and Welsh National Assembly will have some impact on the making of health policy. In Scotland, the issue will be about needing to maintain a separate Scottish NHS but the Parliament will also be seen as providing a new forum for debating the public's health which, despite expenditure some 22% above the UK average, is generally worse than in the rest of the UK. In Wales, the Assembly has already set itself a task to become more involved in health issues, especially in relation to increasing public accountability and examining community health needs. At the time of writing, it is not clear what impact the Northern Ireland Assembly will have on health policy but increasing sub national determination is bound to shift an emphasis towards Belfast. In future, therefore, despite the existence of a national health service, we may see more diversity between countries in the UK.

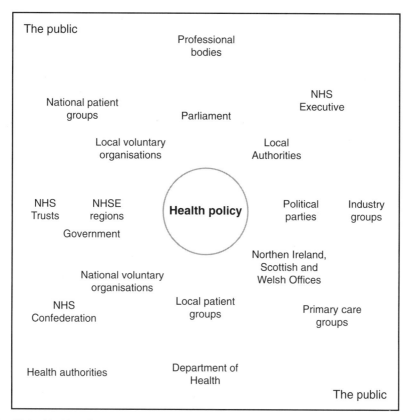

The public

Professional
bodies

National patient
groups

NHS
Executive

Parliament

Local voluntary
organisations

Local
Authorities

NHS   NHSE
Trusts   regions

Health policy

Political
parties

Industry
groups

Government

Northen Ireland,
Scottish and
Welsh Offices

National voluntary
organisations

NHS
Confederation

Local patient
groups

Primary care
groups

Health authorities

Department of
Health

The public

Fig. 13.1   Health policy network.

Local frameworks

Recent changes in primary care organisation and the recognition of the public health role of community nursing have provided more opportunities for nurses to become engaged in public health policy making at the local level. There is also a growing awareness of the important role that community nurses play in developing local contacts with community, user and voluntary groups such as play groups, community health groups, service user groups and community health forums. Turton et al argued in Chapter 11 that local public health action has an important contribution to make to improving public health and a number of studies have identified the enormous range of activity that this encompasses (Peckham et al 1996, Lazenbatt 1997). However, it is important to recognise that local action involves a variety of organisational and locational contexts.

The key public health policy makers at a local level are health and local authorities. Neither is a simple unified organisation but represents a mixture of professional and managerial groupings. Health authorities have formal responsibility for developing public health strategy in collaboration with local authorities. In terms of formal policy making, these agencies have the key role of developing health improvement programmes (HIPs) and setting public health targets. While there are some slight differences between English, Northern Irish, Scottish and Welsh health structures, the importance of the health authority or board in this instance is the same. However, there are some important differences in structure in Northern Ireland where there are joint health and social services boards and, as indicated above, in the future the Welsh Assembly is likely to take on some important strategic health policy roles which are bound to impact on public health policy. Health authorities are responsible to the board which is made up of executive directors of the HA together with non-executive directors appointed by the Secretary of State for Health. Thus the mechanisms are highly centralised. However, as will be explored later in this chapter, there are significant opportunities for nurses to become involved in local public health policy making. Before doing this, it is useful to explore the national context of public health policy.

THE BASIS OF CURRENT HEALTH-CARE POLICY

In the 1990s central government policy in relation to the NHS was focused upon the development of purchasing, particularly fundholding and total purchasing (EL(94)79). There were alternative primary care-based approaches to purchasing, such as GP and locality commissioning, but up until the end of 1995, these had failed to receive recognition by the government. With regard to public health, the main policy was the *Health of the nation* (DoH 1992a) which essentially ignored the findings of previous reports on structural influences on health and in particular the Black and Whitehead reports on inequality and health (Townsend 1980, Whitehead 1988). The previous government had also remained a less than enthusiastic supporter of Health for All (HFA) and, as Ranade (1994) has argued:

...the prospects for local action were constrained by the government's lack of political commitment to, or even understanding of, HFA's principles and prerequisites. Indeed, the thrust of public policy and the ideology of Thatcherism were antithetical to these principles ... (p. 141)

Key changes in the previous government's policy towards primary care emerged in late 1995 and early 1996 with the acceptance of a variety of primary care-led approaches to purchasing and an emphasis on the provision of primary care services. The government conducted a 'listening exercise' which led to the publishing of an NHSE working paper (NHSE 1996) at the beginning of the summer of 1996 and two White Papers later the same year (DoH 1996a,b). These documents opened a debate about primary care delivery, the organisation of primary care and what its role in purchasing should be. Part of the government's proposals included the establishment of primary care pilot projects to explore alternative approaches to contracting for general medical and general dental services (DoH 1996a, Appendix A). These White Papers provided for the basis for the NHS (Primary Care) Act 1997 which was passed with cross-party support in March 1997.

Key changes in public health policy were beginning to emerge in 1995, with the publication of a paper on health inequalities under the *Health of the nation* (DoH 1995a) programme clearly signalling a change in the government's view on the causes of ill health. However, the focus was on what response the NHS could make to health inequalities rather than a broad approach across all government policy areas. This led to a range of work on health inequalities (Centre for Reviews and Dissemination 1995), including a major DoH research and development programme, and preempted the current government's review of health inequalities in the Acheson Report (DoH 1998a).

During the 1970s there was also a growing debate about the principles of health visiting following the move from local to health authority provision. This culminated in the statement of principles of health visiting by the Council for the Education and Training of Health Visitors (CETHV) which firmly placed health visiting in a wider public health model (CETHV 1977). In many ways this was a rediscovery of the public health nursing role which underpinned the early development of community nursing (Ottewill & Wall 1990). Little further work on the public health contribution of nursing was undertaken in the 1980s but with the introduction of purchasing in the 1990s, there was a renewed interest in relation to purchasing, especially in health needs assessment. Following the publication of the *Health of the nation* (DoH 1992a), the DoH provided guidance on the role of nurses, midwives and health visitors in promoting health, again stressing the broader public health role. However, it was in 1995, with the publication of *Making it happen* (SNMAC 1995), that the public health role of nurses achieved more formal recognition. Despite the formal recognition there was still little guidance on implementation or how the public health role should be integrated into purchasing and commissioning at health authority and primary care levels.

Political influence on current public health policy

The election of the Labour government in May 1997 appeared to herald a change in emphasis for health-care policy. Within weeks of the election, the government had appointed the UK's first Minister for Public Health and announced the end of the internal market with a shift towards more collaborative arrangements for health-care commissioning and provision.

The blueprint for the new NHS came with key White Papers in England, Northern Ireland, Scotland and Wales (DoH 1997, Northern Ireland Office 1997, 1998, Scottish Office 1998, Welsh Office 1998). The common theme to these White Papers was the abolition of the internal market and GP fundholding and a move towards partnerships and collaboration. However, the reforms were not to sweep away all the vestiges of the internal market as health authorities were to remain purchasers and hospitals and community trusts would remain as provider organisations. The main new organisational change is the introduction of primary care groups (PCGs) in England and Northern Ireland (local health groups in Wales) which are integrated commissioning/providing organisations grouping together a number of GPs and their practices. In Scotland the reforms are taking a different path with unified community and primary care trusts but with the commissioning role retained within the health boards.

Public health policy was the subject of a Green Paper *Our healthier nation* (DoH 1998b) published in early 1998. This set out the government's agenda for public health for consultation prior to the production of a White Paper later in the year setting out the government's policy intentions. However, public health policy is not simply restricted to *Our healthier nation* and key developments have also been put forward in the White Paper on food and nutrition establishing the Food Standards Agency (DoH 1998c) and more recently in the White Paper on tobacco (DoH 1998d). *The new NHS* also identified public health policy developments with HIPs and health action zones (HAZs). In addition, the Green Paper on public health outlines proposals for the establishment of healthy living centres which will develop a more multidisciplinary and community approach to primary care.

While the White and Green Papers can be seen as presenting a fundamentally new framework for health policy, there are clear continuities between current policy thinking and developments prior to 1997. As suggested above, many elements of the post-1991 NHS reforms are to remain and the creation of PCGs can be seen as an inevitable development of GP commissioning which expanded in a number of guises in the mid-1990s. Changes in Conservative government policy were clearly visible with the publication of the two White Papers on primary care in 1996 (DoH 1996a,b) and the passing of the NHS (Primary Care) Act 1997 which paved the way for the Primary Care Act pilots (PCAPS) and GP commissioning pilots. In particular, the experience of multipractice purchasing including GP commissioning, multifunds and total purchasing pilots can be seen to have had a significant impact on central policy development and the concept of PCGs.

Common policy themes

Collaboration and participation are emphasised within both the Green and White Papers. These ideas come together in proposals for healthy living centres to be funded from the Lottery and are also evident in the proposals for HAZs. The development of HAZs represents one element of the government's intention to provide 'joined up solutions' to complex problems, a desire to move away from the compartmentalism which characterises health and social care issues. Collaboration between health and local authorities is also highlighted as essential to the broader promotion of public health and the proposals for HIPs (DoH 1997) emphasise the important role of local authorities.

Direct involvement in the development of HIPs is seen as a key task for local authorities and will be underpinned by a new statutory duty to 'improve the economic, social and environmental well-being of their areas' (DoH 1998b) and the Green Paper envisages an important role for local authorities in tackling public health issues through housing, transport, education and social policies. Therefore the proposals contained in the Green Paper support a wider public health approach and implicitly acknowledge the primary care function of other front-line agencies and their importance in improving health. This approach was echoed in the Chief Medical Officer's report on public health (DoH 1998e) published shortly after *Our healthier nation*.

However, responsibility for the coordination of the public health strategy will remain with the directors of public health at regional and health authority level. Health authorities are still dominated by the medical model, raising concerns that the ever-present need to increase the provision of medical services may override the longer term strategic need to develop collaborative strategies. Another concern is that there appear to be few links between the White Paper on the NHS and the Green Paper on public health. So, while the rhetoric of collaboration and partnership may be present in both NHS and public health policy, the mechanisms for implementation of policy do not appear to be thought through.

Both the White and Green Papers also support a shift towards a population-based approach rather than an individual patient-centred one. Ham (1996) has argued that the experience of purchasing and commissioning in the mid-1990s led to a view that improvements to health care could be achieved by combining patient-centred and population-focused approaches to purchasing. The development of PCGs continues this concept by fusing a practice-based patient focus with an area-based population focus. How well these two approaches can be blended together is not known as the results of the total purchasing pilots (TPP) evaluation do not really provide a clear picture (Mays et al 1998). However, the TPP study and other research do suggest that some form of localised approach together with an individual focus can lead to some improvements in health-care services such as improved outpatient procedures, better and faster histology services and closer GP/clinician collaboration (Le Grand et al 1998).

It is interesting, though, that despite the prominence given to the development of primary care in the White Paper on the NHS, there is little reference to the role of PCGs in the Green Paper on public health. The role of HIPs is referred to only with regard to their responsibility for '... planning and developing services for smaller populations that will be sensitive to local health needs' (pp. 48–49) and as one of the health partners in HAZs (p. 51). Their role appears to continue to be based in medical care rather than the broader perspective of health.

The White Paper primarily focuses on the underpinning of medical knowledge and the role of the doctor in its proposals for PCGs. This does not sit easily with a more participative approach and certainly provides the potential for a more medically dominated framework to health-care services. In this context, it is of concern that the proposed performance framework for the new NHS remains disease based which will influence the measurement of health outcomes. In contrast, the Green Paper argues for a broader approach to health with its inclusion of a range of statutory, private and voluntary agencies in tackling public health.

Continuity and change in health policy

Klein (1995) has argued that while there were significant changes to the NHS in 1991 there was also a large element of continuity with the past, as some aspects of the change within the NHS were constrained by existing structures, past experience and the politically possible. For example, the NHS remained free at the point of use, it remained universal and is still funded by taxation. At the same time, there were enormous organisational changes which have altered the fabric of the NHS, including the creation of the internal market, independent provider trusts and GP fundholding. Yet these changes would not have been possible without the introduction of general management and the experience of the Resource Management Initiative in the 1980s (Klein 1995). Thus, we can see that continuity is an important element of policy development.

As argued above, there are key elements of current policy which build on changes in the 1990s. Some of these are broad policy changes which have developed over the past two or three decades. For example, the development of primary care has been a continuing theme since the mid-1960s which saw the introduction of the Family Doctor's Charter and attempts in the 1970s and 1980s to improve the quality of general practice (Peckham et al 1998). This historical development, together with the initial establishment of GPs as independent practitioners, has shaped the pattern of primary care in the UK and provided a legacy which the current government is having to address. In particular, PCGs have been structured around general practice and in 1997 the need for government to provide guarantees of independence to GPs dominated debates around the establishment of PCGs. The development of PCGs also had important implications for nursing as the inclusion of primary care nurses on PCG boards was a significant development but these debates received less attention. Other key themes of lasting relevance in health-care policy are centralisation/decentralisation, professionalism/managerialism and accountability.

Centralisation versus decentralisation

A direct result of the 1991 reforms was the greater fragmentation of the NHS. It was originally established as a centrally coordinated service in 1948 but the internal market created more independent health authority purchasers, independent provider trusts and GP fundholders. The adoption of the internal market created a new framework for decision making with more local strategy development. However, not all central control was relinquished as the Health of the nation established national health targets and in 1994 regions were brought within the NHSE.

One of the key aims of the White Paper *The new NHS* is to develop a one-nation health service. The government is keen to remove inequities in treatment and standards of service between different areas. The establishment of national service frameworks, the National Institute for Clinical Effectiveness to advise on best practice and the Commission for Health Improvement to act as a service standards body are national approaches to addressing these issues. At the same time, the number of purchasing and commissioning bodies is being reduced from some 3600 bodies in 1997 to 481 PCGs. These attempts at reducing fragmentation and increasing central standards may, however, be at odds with the development of strong independent PCGs which are more decentralist in approach. Thus there will be a continued tension between the desire for localised commissioning to meet local needs and the need to ensure that central NHS goals and unified standards are achieved.

Similarly, within its proposals for public health the government has raised the issues of the need for central targets but with the development of local objectives. The range of targets has been simplified compared to the Health of the nation and it has been suggested that health authorities develop local targets. For example, the national sexual health targets have been abolished and health authorities will set these based on local needs. However, sexual health remains an area of political controversy and while national targets have not been set for teenage pregnancy, the government is developing a national framework. In fact, the whole basis of *Our healthier nation* is of a contract between central government, local areas and individuals. In this sense the government has acknowledged the need to address local/national tensions. What is missing as yet are the mechanisms for achieving a balance between what are often competing local and national priorities.

Managerialism

The new NHS also represents a further extension of managerialism within the UK health service with the incorporation of primary care more firmly within the NHS. The development of PCGs sets out an agenda for incorporating primary care within the NHS hierarchy and presents a real challenge to the independent nature of general practice. The organisation of commissioning is likely to lead to greater managerial scrutiny of and accountability for primary care. Yet at the same time, the White Paper promotes the development of clinical governance and supports the increased involvement of clinicians and others, such as nurses, in service planning and commissioning. This support for clinical involvement is a key theme of the White Paper and appears to encourage professional involvement in decision making which may be at odds with increasing managerial control.

At one level, this emphasis on professional involvement is to be welcomed as there is a shift away from a specific focus on doctors to an increased nursing role in decision making, particularly in PCGs. However, there is still a clear preference for doctors to be lead clinicians in both commissioning and clinical governance as nurses have less representation on PCG boards. However, it is not clear that clinical skills are necessarily the most appropriate skills for commissioning and there is a tension between whether nurses in managerial roles would be more suitable nursing representatives than those with only clinical experience.

Clinical accountability

This dominance of the clinical professional is also important when considering accountability. Although the NHS has traditionally been viewed as being held accountable centrally through the Secretary of State for Health, in reality accountability has always been something of a patchwork quilt with management and organisational structures using different accountability mechanisms for clinical and nursing staff who have their own professional bodies. In addition, there is also the Health Service Ombudsman, whose remit covers dealing with instances of maladministration, and community health councils (CHCs) who have provided some sense of local accountability. It must be recognised, however, that the centralised political accountability has provided the key focus of attention, as exemplified by crises in service provision in the 1990s to which various Secretaries of State felt the need to respond. These included the problems with the London Ambulance Service, supervision of people in the community with mental health problems, clinical incompetence and cases of fraud and probity of board members and NHS staff.

Key to the debates within the NHS during the early part of the 1990s was the extent to which the market mechanism could provide an appropriate route for accountability and how traditional routes of accountability through management and professional structures could be maintained in a fragmented NHS. These debates have been superseded to some extent by the White Paper which places a substantial emphasis on a public service ethos and public accountability. However, there is little detail on how this public accountability will be achieved – an issue of particular concern to PCGs. They must be accountable to the public but traditionally general practice has been largely unaccountable to both the NHS and the public.

This is of particular concern to community staff who may see their jobs transferred to general practice. Clearly PCGs will have to meet financial and administrative criteria and targets set by the NHSE and their health authority but who will monitor the level of care, types of care provided and decisions made within the PCG and the practices? The 1995 NHSE GP fundholding accountability document has been used as the basis for developing a PCG accountability framework but little progress has been made on developing adequate accountability mechanisms for primary care (Klein & New 1998, Lupton et al 1998).

There are also significant questions to be answered with regard to clinical accountability. While the reforms have made clinicians more accountable to their employing organisations and to other clinicians, their accountability to patients has not been strengthened. The Patient's Charters (DoH 1992b, 1995b) do provide a definitive level of standards but these do not relate to quality of care and do not confer any substantial rights. For example, the Charter right to information is limited by a clinician's freedom to decide what information to give. The Patient Partnership initiative (NHSE 1996) has also underpinned developments in promoting patient involvement in clinical decision making and this is an area where further developments are likely with increasing provision of health information directly to patients and a shift in power within clinical consultations away from the clinician to the patient. This has important consequences for clinical practice but also may offer nurses increased roles in relation to supporting patient information services and working with user groups.

Following the 1991 reforms, there were concerns about the increasing secretiveness of the NHS (Longley 1993): Secretive trust boards, fewer DHA/FHSA meetings, smaller boards and the demise of regions resulting in the loss of regional boards. There was some discussion that CHCs could have been funded directly by the NHSE. The Labour government has taken steps to arrest this drift toward secretiveness and NHS provider board meetings must now be held in public. However, there is still a serious concern over what the most appropriate role for CHCs should be and the debate about how they are funded and what they do is still rumbling on.

Perhaps the most unknown factor is how public accountability through consumer and community involvement will develop. Current pressure to achieve responsiveness to consumers and the emphasis on developing charter-type standards are clearly creating a different environment within the NHS. There is much discussion about appropriate mechanisms for achieving involvement in health care, particularly those aspects of purchasing which create fierce debate such as the rationing or prioritising of health care (Lupton et al 1998). To date, these debates have centred around the health authority. In future, the focus will shift to PCGs which lack any history in this area of work and which are dominated by GPs who are not renowned for working in collaborative and participative ways.

Current policy and public health nursing

For nursing, the SNMAC report *Making it happen* remains the key guiding policy document. However, PCGs and the proposals set out in Our healthier nation provide a new framework for public health nursing. In addition, the Primary Care Act pilots have also provided opportunities for extending nursing roles although these are limited and tend to be within an individual patient context.

The 1970s and 1980s saw significant changes in the delivery of community nursing, with the shift from local to health authorities in 1974 and key debates about the development of primary health-care teams based on GP practices rather than areas. Ironically, where the Cumberlege Report (DHSS 1986) failed to shift community nursing policy towards area-based work because of significant GP pressure, the new proposals for PCGs may provide a vehicle for developing area-based work. The drawing of population boundaries and the shift in focus from patients to populations may provide a significant opportunity for the reorganisation of community nursing services away from a narrow practice focus. In fact, such a focus will become increasingly important if PCGs are to develop as population-based commissioners requiring changes in working patterns, involvement in public health activities and the development of a nurse commissioning role. The development of PCGs is also part of a changing local landscape in public health policy within which there may be opportunities for nurses to become more involved in the policy process.

PUBLIC HEALTH POLICY: THE LOCAL POLICY FRAMEWORK

As identified earlier in this chapter, the key agencies responsible for public health at a local level are health authorities and local authorities. Within this basic framework there are, however, key players including public health specialists, environmental health officers and PCGs as well as specific programmes such as Health for All, Agenda 21, HAZs, HIPs and regeneration programmes (SRBS, City Challenge).

Within the health authority the key group are the public health specialists who will lead the development of the HIP. Making contact with your local public health specialists is important in any public health work. The department or group may include a public health nurse and/or other workers adopting community health development approaches. In some areas the public health department also includes health promotion officers although these may also be based in the local community trust. The key roles of the public health department include:

- identifying the health needs of the local population;
- providing clinical support to health authority and PCG commissioners;
- preparing the health authority's HIP in collaboration with formal partners (LAs), PCGs and other local agencies;
- providing policy support to local health authorities on public health issues.

The establishment of PCGs (and their counterparts in the rest of the UK) provides a further local focus for public health activity in the health service. A key role of PCGs (except in Scotland where the health board retains this responsibility) is to commission health-care services on behalf of its population. Nurses have both board-level responsibilities as commissioners, holding one or two of the board places, and operational responsibility within the group for community and practice nursing services. This may present further opportunities in the future for primary care nurses to influence health policy through inputs into the commissioning process and strategic direction of PCGs. This is a new context within which local policy can be developed and given the de facto position of a primary care nurse on the board, it is clear that the government intends that local primary care nurses should have an influence on local commissioning and service development at a local policy level. However, the formal role and involvement of primary care nurses is likely to remain limited given the stronger position of GPs on PCG boards and within the primary health-care team.

Local authorities are generally split into directorates or departments with specific functional roles (e.g. education, housing, social services, environmental health). There are differences between areas as to the organisational arrangements for local government with key functional differences between county, district and unitary authorities. The latter, as their name implies, have responsibility for all local services and can be found mainly in urban areas such as Bristol, Newcastle and Birmingham or where there are strong arguments for a unified local government structure such as on the Isle of Wight. The rest of the country is split into counties and districts with the former holding the more strategic functions such as education, social services and transportation while districts are responsible for more local services such as housing, refuse collection, environmental health and leisure.

The key difference between health and local authorities is their democratic nature. Health authorities and PCGs are part of a national structure with local operational organisation. Accountability is upwards to the NHSE and the Secretary of State for Health who is a member of the Cabinet and responsible to Parliament. In contrast, LAs are local organisations with local democratic accountability through elected councillors. However, the majority of local authority funding comes in the form of grants from central government. In this sense the public sector in the UK is highly centralised. LAs do, however, have a range of functions which relate to public health including environmental health, planning, refuse collection, parks and leisure, housing, social services and transport. In fact, prior to 1974 LAs were responsible for most aspects of community nursing and also for the public health functions now held by HAs (Ottewill & Wall 1990).

While there has been a consistent recognition of the importance of the LA public health role, formal involvement in developing public health strategy with health authorities has been very limited. Developments arising from the *Health of the nation* programme identified the health promotion role of LAs alongside health services and LAs have shown themselves to be strong supporters of the Healthy Cities and Health for All movements. However, the Green Paper on public health and the Chief Medical Officer's report on the public health function (DoH 1998e) have formally recognised the importance of LA/HA collaboration on public health strategy and action. The development of urban regeneration has also been acknowledged as being important for addressing local health issues. New single regeneration bids (SRBs) must identify potential health benefits and health plays an important role within Agenda 21 developments.

Influencing the local public health policy process

Influencing local authorities mirrors the policy networks described earlier in this chapter for the national government. At the local level policy is developed by councils on the advice of their professional officers and local pressure groups, through local political processes, pressure from other organisations (such as health authorities), national policy frameworks and direct central government guidance. It is likely that in future public health policy (specifically the local HIP) will be developed collaboratively. Thus PCGs will become another group of agencies working with local authorities. The HIP will be one of the most important local public health strategic documents and influencing the development of the HIP should be an objective for all local stakeholders, including primary care nurses. The main opportunities for this will be through alliances with professional bodies and local community organisations and formally through the mechanisms of the PCG, community trust and health authority.

Of these, the most important route will be via the PCG not just in terms of the nurse representative on the board but by influencing key stake-holders such as GPs. This can be done at both the practice and PCG levels. The localisation of health care and commissioning does provide a perhaps unique opportunity in the development of the NHS for primary care nurses to actively engage in debates about local public health policy. As is widely recognised, public health is a range of activities and within the PCG there will be opportunities for becoming involved in health needs assessment, health promotion, working with local organisations through SRBs, healthy living centres and health-care commissioning. This will not be an easy road to follow. However, for health visitors and other primary care nurses who already have the key constituents of a public health approach, the introduction of a population focus within primary care will be welcomed despite the fact that in general, the PCG environment may not be public health orientated (Taylor et al 1998; see also Chapter 11).

CONCLUSION

While there would appear to be a degree of continuity between the health policy of the Labour and Conservative governments, central government policy on public health is undergoing important changes from that prevailing in the 1980s and early 1990s. Central to these changes are the acceptance of the need to address health inequalities and the recognition that such inequalities are caused by wider social and environmental problems such as poverty and poor housing. However, despite an emphasis on the need for local agencies to work together, there has been some criticism of the lack of central government policy to directly address these issues. It will take many years before we can tell whether HAZs and healthy living centres have affected people's health. If poverty and income inequalities are the main causes of health inequalities, as argued by Wilkinson (1996), then it is unlikely that these initiatives will have any significant impact, with employment and fiscal policy playing a more central role.

However, there are a number of contexts to public health and health inequalities and improving health-care accessibility for individuals and groups of people currently disadvantaged, improvements to local housing and environments, etc. can have immediate benefits. These activities can be pursued at local levels by working with other agencies or at a national level by supporting and promoting a public health approach to policy development and implementation. Nurses can play a role in these areas of activity. This does require a shift from an operational focus to a more strategic role. However, for many primary care nurses such a role is not new and would be welcomed and, within PCGs, nurses may be the advocates of such an approach and will therefore have an important role in shaping the public health policy of PCGs in the coming years.

REFERENCES

Centre for Reviews and Dissemination 1995 Review of the research on the effectiveness of health service interventions to reduce variations in health. NHS CRD, York
CETHV 1977 An investigation into the principles of health visiting. Council for Education and Training of Health Visitors, London
DHSS 1971 National Health Service reorganisation: a consultative document. DHSS, London
DHSS 1986 Neighbourhood nursing: a focus for care. HMSO, London
DoH 1992a Health of the nation. HMSO, London
DoH 1992b The patient's charter. HMSO, London
DoH 1995a Health of the nation: variations in health. HMSO, London
DoH 1995b The patient's charter. HMSO, London
DoH 1996a Primary care: choice and opportunity. HMSO, London
DoH 1996b Primary care: delivering the future. HMSO, London
DoH 1997 The new NHS: modern, dependable. Cmd. 3807. HMSO, London
DoH 1998a Report of the Independent Inquiry into Inequalities in Health (Acheson Report). HMSO, London
DoH 1998b Our healthier nation. Cmd. 3857. HMSO, London
DoH 1998c The Food Standards Agency: a force for change. Cmd. 3830. HMSO, London
DoH 1998d Smoking kills – A White Paper on tobacco. Cmd. 4177. HMSO, London
DoH 1998e Chief Medical Officer's project to strengthen the public health function in England. A report of emerging findings. NHS Executive, Leeds
Frenk J 1994 Dimensions of health system reform. Health Policy 27: 19–34
Ham C 1992 Health policy in Britain. Macmillan, London
Ham C 1996 Population centred and patient focused purchasing – the UK experience. Millbank Quarterly 74(2): 191–197
Ham C, Hill M 1984 The policy process in the modern capitalist state. Harvester, Brighton
Harrison S, Wood B 1999 Paper presented to PSA Health Politics Conference, 7–8 January, Oxford
Harrison S, Hunter D J, Pollitt C 1990 The dynamics of British health policy. Unwin Hyman, London
Hennessey D 1997 The shape of things to come. Nursing Times 93(27): 36–38
Klein R 1995 The new politics of the NHS. Longman, London
Klein R, New B 1998 Two cheers? Reflections on the health of NHS democracy. King's Fund, London
Lazenbatt A 1997 Targeting health and social need. The contribution of nurses, midwives and health visitors. Departments of Nursing, University of Ulster and Queen's University of Belfast
LeGrand J, Mays N, Mulligan J 1998 Learning from the NHS internal market. King's Fund, London
Longley D 1993 Public law and health service accountability. Open University Press, Buckingham
Lupton C, Peckham S, Taylor P 1998 Managing public involvement in health care purchasing. Open University Press, Buckingham
Mays N, Good N, Killoran A et al 1998 Total purchasing: a step towards primary care groups. King's Fund, London
Ministry of Health 1962 A hospital plan for England and Wales. Cmnd 1604. HMSO, London
NHSE 1996 Primary care: the future. NHSE, Leeds
Northern Ireland Office 1997 Well into 2000. HMSO, Belfast

Northern Ireland Office 1998 Fit for the future: consultation paper. NI Office, Belfast

Ottewill R, Wall A 1990 The growth and development of the community health services. Business Education Publishers, Newcastle

Peckham S, Macdonald J, Taylor P 1996 Towards a public health model of primary care. Public Health Alliance, Birmingham

Peckham S, Turton P, Taylor P 1998 The missing link. Health Service Journal 108(5606): 22–23

Ranade W 1994 A future for the NHS? Longman, London

Scottish Office 1998 Designed to care: renewing the NHS in Scotland. HMSO, Edinburgh

SNMAC 1995 Making it happen. DoH, London

Spurgeon P 1997 How nurses can influence policy. Nursing Times 5(93):34–35

Taylor P, Peckham S, Turton P 1998 A public health model of primary care: from rhetoric to reality. Public Health Alliance, Birmingham

Townsend P 1980 The Black Report. Penguin, Harmondsworth

Welsh Office 1998 NHS Wales: putting patients first. HMSO, Cardiff

Whitehead M 1988 The health divide. HEA, London

Wilkinson R G 1996 Unhealthy societies: the afflictions of inequality. Routledge, London

Williamson C 1992 Whose standards? Consumer and professional standards in health care. Open University Press, Buckingham

---

FURTHER READING

Baggott R 2000 Politics and policy. Macmillan, London.
This book provides an overview of key policy debates relating to public health and explores many of the main themes currently being debated within the public health field.

Macdonald J 1992 Primary health care. Medicine in its place. Earthscan, London.
This book provides an excellent introduction to the wider concept of primary health care and the limitations of primary medical care. It discusses what is needed to achieve public health within a primary health-care framework.

Taylor P, Peckham S, Turton P 1998 A public health model of primary care: from concept to reality. Public Health Alliance, Birmingham.
An up-to-date account of key developments in primary care and public health with a wealth of discussion about problems and issues in practice.

Curtis S, Taket A 1996 Health and societies. Arnold, London.
This text provides an excellent introduction to the geography of health, health inequalities, public health and policy making with an international perspective.

Ham C 1992 Health policy in Britain. The politics and organisation of the National Health Service, 3rd edn. Macmillan, Basingstoke.
This is a classic on the policy-making process in the NHS. The third edition is somewhat out of date but Professor Chris Ham is working on an updated edition.

Green J, Thorogood N 1998 Analysing health policy. A sociological approach. Longman, London.
For a rather different perspective on health policy, perhaps with a critical eye on recent changes, this book will be of interest. The authors take a more sociological approach to health policy and cover issues such as public health and health promotion, equity, primary care and issues of professionalism and managerialism.

Useful addresses

Association for Public Health/Public Health Alliance
138 Digbeth
Birmingham B5 6DR
Tel: 0121 643 7628
Fax: 0121 643 4541
(Has Welsh and Scottish groups)

Community Practitioners and Health Visitors Association
50 Southwark Street
London SE1 1UN
Tel: 020 7378 7255

CPHVA in Scotland
94 Constitution Street
Leith
Edinburgh EH6 6AW

Faculty of Public Health Medicine
4 St Andrews Place
Regents Park
London NW1 4LB
Tel: 020 7935 0243
Open to medically qualified doctors training to be or practising as public health physicians.

Friends of the Earth
26–28 Underwood Street
London N1 7JQ
Tel: 020 7490 1555

Health Education Authority
Trevelyan House
30 Great Peter Street
London SW1P 2HW
Tel: 020 7222 5300

Health Education Board for Scotland
Woodburn House
Canaan Lane
Edinburgh EH10 45G
Tel: 0131 536 5500
Fax: 0131 536 5501
Email: hebsweb@hebs.scot.nhs.uk

Health Promotion Agency for Northern Ireland
18 Ormeau Avenue
Belfast BT2 8HS
Tel: 028 9031 1611
Fax: 028 9031 1711

Health Promotion Wales
Ffynnon-las
Ty Glas Avenue
Llanishen
Cardiff CF4 5DZ

National Community Health Resource
57 Chalton St
London NW1 1HU
Tel: 020 7383 3841

National Dental Health Education Group
25 Ash Grove
Stratford Upon Avon
Warks CV37 0DR

National Energy Action
St Andrew's House
90–92 Pilgrim Street
Newcastle-upon-Tyne NE1 6SG
Tel: 0191 261 5677

National Food Alliance
2nd Floor
94 White Lion Street
London N1 9PF
Tel: 020 7837 1228

Office for Public Health in Scotland
1 Lilybank Gardens
Glasgow G12 8R2

Royal College of Nursing
20 Cavendish Square
London WIM 0AB
Tel: 020 7409 3333
(The College has professional groupings for registered health visitors and
other community nurse groups.)

Royal Institute of Public Health
3 Birdcage Walk
London SW1H 9JH

Sustrans
35 King Street
Bristol BS1 4DX
Tel: 0117 926 8893

Index